W9-DHS-084

DR. TAYLOR'S SELF-HELP MEDICAL GUIDE

❦

Robert B. Taylor, M.D.

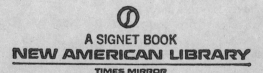
A SIGNET BOOK
NEW AMERICAN LIBRARY
TIMES MIRROR

Publisher's Note

The ideas, procedures, and suggestions contained in this book are not intended as a substitute for consulting with your physician. All matters regarding your health require medical supervision.

NAL BOOKS ARE AVAILABLE AT QUANTITY DISCOUNTS WHEN USED TO PROMOTE PRODUCTS OR SERVICES. FOR INFORMATION PLEASE WRITE TO PREMIUM MARKETING DIVISION, THE NEW AMERICAN LIBRARY, INC., 1633 BROADWAY, NEW YORK, NEW YORK 10019.

A hardcover edition of this book is published by Atheneum Publishers. The hardcover editions was published simultaneously in Canada by McClelland and Stewart Ltd.

 SIGNET TRADEMARK·REG. U.S. PAT. OFF. AND FOREIGN COUNTRIES REGISTERED TRADEMARK—MARCA REGISTRADA HECHO EN CHICAGO, U.S.A.

SIGNET, SIGNET CLASSICS, MENTOR, PLUME, MERIDIAN AND NAL BOOKS *are published by The New American Library, Inc., 1633 Broadway, New York, New York 10019*

FIRST SIGNET PRINTING, JULY, 1978

5 6 7 8 9 10 11 12

PRINTED IN THE UNITED STATES OF AMERICA

IS YOUR FAMILY SPENDING HUNDREDS OF DOLLARS A YEAR ON UNNECESSARY DOCTOR BILLS?

Millions of Americans pay for the doctor when all they need is plain and simple information about everyday ailments that trouble them. Most people don't know how to recognize, let alone treat, these illnesses. Now an experienced family physician cuts through the clinical jargon and explains how the layman can detect—and often cure—more than 200 familiar complaints, from acne and animal bite to warts and whooping cough. In each case, he tells exactly what you must do to help yourself, and exactly when you must abandon self-help and turn to the professionals. He prescribes home treatments, lists nonprescription drugs by brand name, describes scores of legitimate natural remedies that you can prepare in your kitchen, and, most important, he gives invaluable tips for preventing these maladies in the first place. This all-inclusive home medical guide is a must for every family seeking overall health protection.

DR. ROBERT B. TAYLOR grew up in Monongahela, Pa., attended Bucknell, and got his M.D. in 1961 at Temple University School of Medicine. After serving three years at the U.S. Public Health Service Hospital in Norfolk, Va., he started up a bustling family practice in New Paltz, N.Y. A charter diplomate of the American Board of Family Practice and a charter fellow of the American Academy of Family Physicians, Dr. Taylor has written three medical texts as well as two popular health handbooks, *Feeling Alive after 65* and *Dr. Taylor's Guide to Healthy Skin for All Ages.*

SIGNET Medical Books
for Your Reference Shelf

Contents

Preface

Today's medical techniques, drugs, and appliances eclipse the wildest dreams of our ancestors; but with the advances in medicine have come rising costs and shrinking availabiltiy of health care. Few of us can afford the twenty-five-dollar (or more) consultation fee to have a low-back strain treated by an orthopedic specialist or have an internist direct therapy of the flu. Nor is such consultation often necessary, since these everyday ailments and hundreds more can be treated at home—if only you know how!

Case Report

Sarah S., age 23, suffered a hacking cough, nasal congestion, and a fever of 100.4°F. She visited her local physician, who prescribed 30-mg pseudoephedrine tablets (Sudafed) four times daily, an expectorant containing glyceryl guaiacolate and dextromethorphan (Robitussin DM Syrup), and advice concerning rest and fluids.

The cost of treating Sarah's cold was:

Doctor's office call	$15.00
Prescription Medication:	
Sudafed Tablets	4.25
Robitussin DM	3.75
	$23.00

If Sarah had only known, the same treatment was available for much less. Her unnecessary expenses were a $15 doctor's fee and $1.75 pharmacist's fee added to the retail cost of each of two prescriptions for drugs available over the counter. The cost of treatment should have been:

Sudafed Tablets	$2.50
Robitussin DM	2.00
	$4.50

Most of us enjoy good health, but almost no one has super-health—freedom from all minor ailments. At any given time, the average individual (you or I) suffers a half dozen minor ailments: dandruff, sinus congestion, varicose veins, cold sores, headache, constipation, and on and on. Medical consultation might be enlightening, but it's likely that the physician will prescribe therapy that needs no written prescription: the doctor's diet, exercise, shampoo, laxative, moist-heat treatment, or what-have-you is often available without prescription—if you understand the disease and its treatment. On the other hand, the patient whose disorder demands medical consultation gets the most from his doctor visit when he has done his homework, studying his symptoms, possible causes, and current treatment.

This book helps you chart a course to better health. Within these pages you'll learn how to:

- Cope with minor ailments through diet, exercise, physical therapy, nonprescription medication, and natural remedies.
- Recognize when a medical problem is beyond the scope of self-help care.
- Find public and private agencies that take a special interest in specific diseases, including addresses to which you can write for guidance and help.
- Evaluate the quality of medical care you receive.

Self-help medical care can spell the difference between ho-hum health and physical fitness, while saving money that would be spent for professional treatment of trivial complaints. It can spare the hassle of office calls, x-rays, blood tests, and insurance forms—all for ailments you could treat at home.

Acknowledgements

The most I can do for my friend is simply to be his friend.

Henry David Thoreau, *Journal*
February 7, 1841

The nonfiction writer needs up-to-the-minute facts, ready references, artistic assistance, the creative urge, time to complete the task, and friends who understand.

Now that the last manuscript page has been typed and proofread, I have time to look out the window at the mountains and reflect on all those who shared in preparation of this book.

Bouquets and friendship go to:

typist Carol Ostmark
artist Karin Blake
pharmaceutical advisors Robert Van Vlack and Ira Bomze
my office staff—Hazel Kowalik, R.N. and Mary Ellen Rebhan
my parents—Mr. and Mrs. O. C. Taylor
    and to
Sharon, Diana, and Anita

Author's Note

Doctor Taylor's Self-Help Medical Guide is intended to serve as a reference source describing the diagnosis and treatment of many ailments, common and uncommon. Since most ailments are known by several names, the reader looking for information concerning a specific illness should first consult the index.

The facts and opinions contained herein are presented for informational purposes only, rather than as specific therapeutic recommendations for the individual reader or patient. The book is intended to supplement, not to replace, periodic health checkups and necessary medical consultation with the physician.

The Common Ailments
of Mankind

ABRASION

Synonyms: scrape, brushburn

Mary's bicycle slides on loose gravel and she falls, landing on an elbow. Tearfully, she seeks medical care from the family's ever-present medical consultant—Mom.

The abrasion, usually occurring when the skin over a bony prominence, such as the elbow or knee, meets a rough surface such as concrete, scrapes away the outer layer of skin (epidermis), causing burning pain and small bleeding points. Tiny bits of dirt are often imbedded and can cause infection if not removed.

Treatment

The abrasion should first be washed with lots of soap and water. A good choice is pHisoDerm, a sudsing emollient skin cleanser. Rinse copiously with water, then search for tiny imbedded dirt particles, using a magnifying glass and good illumination. Particles can be scraped away delicately, using a cotton-tipped applicator (Q-tip), or, if necessary, picked out with forceps (tweezers).

When Mary's scraped elbow is as clean as can be, disinfect using povidone-iodine (Betadine) solution. Allow the povidone-iodine to dry and, by this time, bleeding should have ceased. Abrasions heal best if left open to the air; they tend to remain moist if covered. However, sometimes the abrasion occurs in an area destined to be exposed to dirt (such as on a child's hand), and common sense decrees that it should be covered; use a Telfa Pad to avoid sticking. If bandaged, the abrasion should be redressed daily—more often if the dressing becomes wet or dirty.

How about a tetanus booster? It's unnecessary in superficial abrasions if Mary has had a tetanus shot within the past five years. However, if the abrasion seems particularly deep and contains one or more puncture wounds, then you should ask the physician about a tetanus booster if Mary's shot record fails to show one within the past year.

Most abrasions heal uneventfully within a few weeks. Dark pigmentation of the skin may persist for several months, but fades with time. The chief danger of the abrasion is infection (signaled by redness, heat, drainage, and increasing pain), which is treated with warm saline soaks followed by the application of Bacitracin Ointment four times daily, perhaps supplemented by an oral antibiotic prescribed by the doctor.

ABSCESS

Synonyms: boil, furuncle

An abscess is a deep skin infection usually caused by the staphylococcus germ. It begins as bacteria enter a scrape in the skin or find a haven in a tiny hair follicle. The germs multiply rapidly, forming a pocket of pus that eventually "points" toward the surface. Local pain, swelling, and redness are present, and the soft pocket of pus can be felt beneath the skin. Sometimes infected lymph glands are found, involving the underarm if the infection is on the wrist or hand, or in the groin with an abscess of the leg or foot.

Treatment

Warm moist compresses draw pus to the surface; salt water (one teaspoonful of table salt in one pint of water about as hot as your bath water) is often used. Alternatively, a good natural compress can be made from onions, papaya, or grated raw potatoes applied directly and covered with a warm, moist 4×4-inch gauze pad.

Draining the pus is the key to successful abscess treatment. This means an incision must be made, allowing pus to escape and relieving painful pressure. A tiny abscess can be drained at home, using a needle cleansed with alcohol; don't worry excessively about sterility since the area is already infected. A larger abscess will require a sharp blade, either the scalpel in the doctor's office or a similar surgically clean cutting edge at home—depending upon the size of the abscess and availability of local medical care.

Following surgical incision, a large abscess is packed with a drain for two or three days to keep the wound open and encourage further drainage of pus. The doctor uses a special gauze packing about ¼-inch wide, and abscesses large enough to require packing are best treated by the physician. When self-help treatment is indicated, however, a small rubber band cleansed with alcohol and inserted in the incision can make a good drain. Be sure to leave an end protruding so that the drain can be grasped for removal 48 hours later.

After the drain is removed, begin soaking, using the warm saline solution described above. Soak the area, using a clean moist gauze pad, half an hour, four times daily. After soaking, apply Bacitracin Ointment and cover with a bulky dressing to absorb pus.

A huge abscess that involves nearby tissues and even regional lymph glands calls for antibiotic treatment, perhaps with penicillin or erythromycin. Such an extensive infection should be treated in the doctor's office.

ACNE

Synonym: acne vulgaris

Acne, terror of the teen-age years, is something the self-help medical therapist can really get his teeth into. There's a vast array of treatments available for simple acne, most costing little and requiring no prescription.

Acne begins when oily secretions plug pores and the sebaceous glands, which supply oil to the skin and hair, continue to produce their fatty sebum. Blackheads form when the opening to the surface is plugged by dark sebum; whiteheads, when a film of skin and sebum blocks the pore; and pimples, when the blocked oil glands become inflamed, balloon, and sometimes burst.

Treatment

Diet plays a role in acne, although its significance is debated by dermatologists. Greasy foods fuel the oil factories, and there's truth to mother's warning that candy causes pimples. To prevent and treat acne, the following foods should be avoided:

Cake and pie
Candy
Chocolate
Fried foods
French fries and potato chips
Iodized salt
Nuts
Salad oil
Soft drinks
Sugar-coated cereals
Syrup

Skin cleansing is the backbone of acne treatment. Excessive skin oils must be removed two or three times daily, leaving the epidermis feeling a little dry. The choice of skin cleanser depends upon your skin texture. We'll consider alternatives, beginning with the mildest first:

- Purpose Hypoallergenic Soap contains salts of fatty acid and glycerin. It's free of harsh detergents and is intended for mild acne on supersensitive skin.
- Cetaphil Lipid-free Skin Cleanser contains sodium lauryl sulfate, propylene glycol, parabens, and alcohol. It's a little stronger than Purpose Soap, but still quite mild for ordinary teen-age acne.
- Seba-Nil contains polysorbate, acetone, and alcohol, and is available in towelettes—use a pad to wipe oily skin areas two or three times daily. Seba-Nil Cleanser is moderately strong and it works well for many youngsters with moderately severe acne.
- Fostex Skin Clenser contains sulfur, salicylic acid, cleansers, and wetting agents. A once-nightly scrub is usually sufficient when supplemented by a once or twice-daily facial with Ivory Soap.

- Benoxyl Lotion, containing benoxyl peroxide, is available in half strength (Benoxyl-5) and full strength (Benoxyl-10). This peeling agent strips away surface oils and leaves the skin feeling rough and dry. Apply to the face one to three times daily to treat well-entrenched acne or nonsensitive skin.
- Retin-A brand of Vitamin A acid is the strongest peeling agent available, and a prescription is required. Retin-A comes in foil-covered saturated swabs or as a liquid; apply to the skin once daily at bedtime—or less often if skin irritation develops. The prescribing physician will caution against mixing Retin-A with compounds containing salicylic acid, sulfur, benzoyl peroxide, or resorcinol, as well as exposing the skin to sunlight or ultraviolet irradiation.
- Brāsivol Scrub Cleanser is available for those who find peeling agents not strong enough and who want to virtually scrub their acne away. Brāsivol Scrub Cleanser contains fused aluminum oxide scrubbing particles in a mixture of neutral soap and surfactant cleansers, and comes in rough, medium, and fine grades. It's intended only for hard-core acne in the toughest skin, and should rarely be a first-choice treatment.

Tetracycline therapy in acne requires a prescription but is usually well worth the trip to the doctor. The antibiotic combats skin bacteria and changes the fatty acid content of sebum. The usual dose is one 250-mg capsule taken twice daily, although the initial dosage may be as high as four a day. Long-term treatment is needed, often for months or years.

Unplugging pores with a comedo extractor (sometimes called a pimple remover) can often hasten acne treatment. Shaped like a tiny spoon with a small central hold (see Figure 1), the comedo extractor is placed over a blackhead, a pimple pointing to the surface, or a whitehead (following a tiny needle puncture). Firm pressure pushes the pore's contents out through the opening. It's really scientific pimple squeezing, and if you have never seen it done it's best to have the family doctor or skin-care specialist show you how.

Ultraviolet light often helps. In the summer the sun can aid self-help acne treatment, drying excessive skin oils. During the winter a sunlamp can be used at home, or perhaps your doctor will prescribe ultraviolet lamp treatments. Some skin-care clinics use the Spectroderm lamp, which dries sebum, opens capillary blood circulation to the skin, and kills surface bacteria.

Hormone therapy is sometimes recommended for teen-age girls with out-of-control acne. Often prescribed as the standard birth control package, the hormone tablets modify sebaceous gland secretions, and can offer dramatic improvement in acne problems of selected patients.

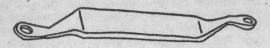

FIGURE 1. *Comedo extractor.*

To overcome acne, you'll need all the information you can get. A good source of self-help is *Doctor Taylor's Guide to Healthy Skin for All Ages* (Arlington House Publishers, New Rochelle, New York), telling the cause and therapy of acne pimples and dozens of other common skin disorders.

ALCOHOL ABUSE

Synonyms: drunkenness, alcoholism

There are nine million American alcoholics—some overt, and others closet drinkers—and alcoholism in a family member blights the life of one of every six persons in the United States. Last year alcoholism contributed to almost three million arrests, 7,000 suicides, 25,000 traffic fatalities, and $15 billion spent in medical care, property damage, and time lost from work. Alcohol abuse is, indeed, a problem of monumental proportions. And it is one medical problem where self-help, with the aid of other afflicted individuals, has a better batting average than medical science.

"Dependent" is the word to describe the alcohol abuser. He's dependent upon other persons—and upon things such as alcohol, cigarettes, and so forth. Usually he's passive, and often a remarkably pleasant individual, posing no threat to those about him. But sometimes affability gives way to depression; or perhaps anger, with destructive behavior, as the alcohol abuser strikes out against society and himself. Unless help is forthcoming, the alcohol abuser may, in the end, form a meaningful relationship only with a bottle.

Taking the Pledge

Self-help may turn the tide against incipient alcohol abuse. Telltale signs that "demon rum" is getting the upper hand include acute anxiety when the liquor stock runs low, the feeling "I can't relax without a drink," and a rising bill at the local liquor store. Eventually comes lying about daily consumption, hiding bottles around the house "in case of emergency," and drinking alone. When these symptoms occur, it's time to stand up and take the pledge.

There is little help available for the alcohol abuser who denies his problem. Step one in self-help is recognizing that liquor threatens to dominate your life. The afflicted individual must say out loud, "I am an alcohol abuser!"

Face the problem, and you have already taken the first and most difficult step in finding a solution.

Step two in the self-help medical therapy of alcohol abuse is resolving not to drink. One jigger of whiskey may be too much, leading to another and another and another. But if you never take the first, there's no problem. Of course, resolving not to drink is easy; keeping your resolution is much harder. As Mark Twain said about smoking, "It's easy to stop. I do it several times a day."

But there are ploys to help keep you on the wagon:

- Remove all liquor from the household. This includes the bottle saved for special occasions, the cooking sherry, and the emergency bottle hidden in the closet.
- Tell the local liquor store: No deliveries to your house, and no sales to you even if you beg.
- At parties, ask for club soda or bitter lemon. If questioned and you hesitate to tell the real reason, blame your stomach, your doctor, or say you are watching your weight.
- Make a bet with your wife (or husband)—something you really don't want to lose. The bet is this: If you can go without a drink for six months, you win. Fail, and you lose the prize.

7

- Shun social functions where temptation may be too strong. Skip the party that always ends with a drinking spree, and stay home and watch TV on New Year's Eve.

The doctor may be some help during the early weeks of abstinence, and this year more than three million alcoholics will seek medical help; perhaps the doctor will prescribe a mild tranquilizer, such as chlordiazepoxide (Librium) or meprobamate (Equanil) to minimize withdrawal symptoms.

Occasionally prescribed is disulfiram (Antabuse), a medication taken daily to deter alcohol ingestion. A drink of alcohol by the individual taking Antabuse is followed by flushing, palpitations, nausea, vomiting, and perhaps unconsciousness. It's a potent medication requiring close supervision by the physician.

Alcoholics Anonymous

The leading self-help organization combating alcoholism, Alcoholics Anonymous, has chapters in every major American city and in almost a hundred other countries. AA defines itself as "a fellowship of men and women who share their experience, strength, and hope with each other that they may solve their common problem and help others to recover from alcoholism."

From a humble beginning in 1935 in Akron, Ohio, AA has built its philosophy upon the firm foundation of self-help, a trust in a Supreme Being, and an instinct for the confidence-building attributes of group therapy. Beginning with the introduction, "I am an alcoholic and it has been five years [or whatever the length of time] since my last drink," the alcoholic describes his experiences in achieving sobriety. Confidence that others have made the grade and a responsibility to those who care help deter taking the next drink.

Information about the local Alcoholics Anonymous chapter is as near as the telephone; AA is listed in the white pages of your telephone directory. Or request information about the nearest chapter by writing:

Alcoholics Anonymous
Box 459

Grand Central Annex
New York, New York 10017

There are affiliate groups for spouses (one-fifth of AA membership is women) and children of alcoholics. For more data write to:

Al-Anon Family Group Headquarters
115 East 23rd Street
New York, New York 10010

Other information is available to individuals and groups who want to learn about alcoholism. Literature and brochures describing services are available from:

National Council on Alcoholism, Inc.
733 Third Avenue
New York, New York 10017

National Council for the Prevention of Alcoholism
6830 Laurel Street, N.W.
Washington, D.C. 20005

AMEBIASIS

Synonym: amebic dysentery

The tiny protozoa Entamoeba histolytica affect about 5 percent of individuals in temperate climates and up to 80 percent of persons living in the tropics. Amoebae, not unlike the amoebae you studied under the microscope in high school biology, infect the intestinal tract, causing cramps and diarrhea. Advanced disease may involve the liver and other organs, making amebiasis a potentially serious problem that demands medical attention.

Preventing Infection

Prevention is the proper thrust of self-help efforts. When traveling always ask, "Is amebiasis a problem in this area?" If so, refuse salads and uncooked vegetables. Soaking uncooked fruits and vegetables in full-strength vinegar (which is really a solution of acetic acid) helps kill any amoebae present; boiling is even better. An experienced world traveler once advised my medical school class, "When traveling in the tropics, never eat uncooked anything that grows below the waist."

Contaminated water can also carry Entamoeba histolytica. Water from the tap should never be consumed unless treated with an aqueous solution of iodine (200 parts per million) or with Halazone tablets (five tablets per quart of water, allowed to stand for 30 minutes). In restaurants, insist upon bottled water and remove the cap yourself. If a waiter brings bottled water with the cap already removed, send it back, since the bottle may have been emptied by a previous (and more astute) traveler and subsequently refilled with tap water. When traveling in the tropics, don't make the mistake of drinking bottled water three meals a day, yet carrying amoebae in your system by rinsing your toothbrush in tap water. And, of course, wash your hands with extra care, as if your health depended upon it. Because it does.

How about preventive medication? Local self-styled experts often recommend one or another drugstore preparation, but leading American authorities discourage the willy-nilly consumption of medication in a vague effort to prevent the various diarrheal diseases of travelers. There's no one drug that works for all, and many of those nostrums readily available in other countries carry the risk of illness as formidable as the disease they are intended to prevent.

Treatment of Amebiasis

Contact a physician promptly if you suspect amebic infection. He will examine a stool specimen, preferably one that is fairly liquid and still warm. If the presence of amebic infection is confirmed, treatment is usually prolonged and will probably involve one or more of the following prescription medications:

> Iodochlorhydroxyquin (Entero-Vioform)
> Diiodohydroxyquin (Diodoquin)
> Arsenical compounds such as Milibis
> Diloxanide furoate (Entamide)
> Emetine bismuth iodide
> Metronidazole (Flagyl)

AMYOTROPHIC LATERAL SCLEROSIS

Synonym: motor system disease

A rare disease usually beginning during the fifth or sixth decade of life, this is a deterioration of the nerves that supply the muscles. Weakness begins in the small muscles of the hands, or perhaps the legs, leading to severe muscle shrinkage (atrophy). The muscles of the eyes are spared and normal alertness is preserved throughout the course of the disease.

Progressive muscular weakness and weight loss are often followed by respiratory paralysis and/or pneumonia. There is no known treatment for amyotrophic lateral sclerosis.

ANAL FISSURE

Synonym: fissure in ano

The anal fissure is a crack in the delicate lining cells of the anus or rectum. Discomfort is usually present and some bleeding may be noted. The cause may be passage of an unusually large bowel movement or irritation due to diarrhea; or no reason for the fissure's presence may be obivous.

Treatment

Self-help medical treatment of the anal fissure includes witch hazel applied on 4 × 4-inch gauze pads. Also useful are Tucks Cotton Flannel Pads, which are saturated with a solution containing 50 percent witch hazel and 10 percent glycerine. After soaking, Medicone Rectal Ointment or Suppositories may be applied. These preparations contain astringent and anesthetic agents, helping to relieve inflammation and close the rectal fissure.

Further recurrences of rectal irritation are minimized by avoiding constipation (taking a mild laxative such as milk of magnesia when necessary) and preventing diarrhea (using Kaopectate to control loose bowel movements). Many individuals with recurrent anal irritation shun toilet tissue and wipe with facial tissue, while others use Tucks Cotton Flannel Pads. A favorite preparation is Balneol Ano-Rectal Cleansing Lotion applied on tissue or cotton, used to cleanse without discomfort after each bowel movement.

Finally, a hot sitz bath (sitting in a tub of hot water) one to three times daily can help ease the discomfort of a rectal fissure.

When to Call the Doctor

Begin to worry about the suspected rectal fissure if bleeding is profuse or persistent. If present for more than a few days, rectal irritation associated with bleeding requires medical examination lest the occasional cancer of this area go undiscovered.

ANEMIA

> She was very anaemic. Her thin lips were pale, and her skin was delicate, of a faint green colour, without a touch of red even in the cheeks.
>
> W. Somerset Maugham
> *Of Human Bondage*

Anemia causes pallor, weakness, and shortness of breath upon exertion. The fingernail beds appear white, there may be dizziness upon standing, and an all-pervading fatigue is usually present.

Iron-Deficiency Anemia

Most anemias are caused by a shortage of iron-rich red blood cells. The question is: Why? And the cause tells whether the anemia is amenable to self-help treatment.

A dietary deficiency of iron is common in infants and elderly individuals, although an iron-poor diet may be eaten at any age. Infants consuming up to one-half gallon of milk each day drink it to the exclusion of iron-containing solid food. These "milk babies" look fat and chubby, but are usually anemic since the milk-rich diet provides little iron.

At the other end of life, oldsters (particularly when living alone) may exist on tea and toast, failing to eat iron-containing meat and vegetables. They too are prone to iron-deficiency anemia.

Even middle-agers may nibble frequently on candy, potato chips, cake, cookies, and milk, failing to consume sufficient dietary iron. All that these individuals need is a daily intake of red meat plus green vegetables, perhaps supplemented by Feosol Tablets or Elixir containing the iron salt ferrous sulfate. The usual adult dose is one to three Feosol Tablets daily, taken with food.

In other instances, iron-deficiency anemia follows blood loss. Here the cause may be elusive and even ominous. Occasionally a woman suffers iron-deficiency anemia following prolonged extra-heavy menstrual flow. The anemia will respond to iron replacement with Feosol Tablets, but she should consult a physician for evaluation and control of a hemorrhagic menstrual flow.

In other individuals the cause may be less obvious. Perhaps there's a bleeding ulcer, dripping blood into the intestinal tract and causing black feces. Or anemia may be the first hint of a cancer of the large intestine. These possibilities underscore the need to have all instances of unexplained anemia investigated by a physician.

Other Anemias

Occurring less commonly are the various other anemias. Yet when they occur, it's important that the correct diagnosis be made, rather than administering iron tablets in a willy-nilly fashion while overlooking the true cause. There is little likelihood of diagnosing the following anemias without medical advice, and the treatment of all requires supervision by the physician:

- Pernicious anemia is a deficiency of Vitamin B_{12} that arrests red blood cells at an immature stage. The youthful blood cells, unable to achieve maturity, lack the oxygen-carrying capacity of their adult counterparts, and cause fatigue, loss of appetite, a distinctive

13

- lemon-yellow skin pallor, and perhaps a staggering gait.
- Mediterranean anemia (thalassemia) is a persistence of a type of hemoglobin that usually disappears from the blood shortly after birth. Sometimes the disease is severe and terminates fatally (thalassemia major), while other individuals carry only the trait (thalassemia minor)—compatible with a normal life.
- Sickle cell anemia, a distinctive disease of blacks, is characterized by muscle and joint pains.
- Hereditary spherocytosis is an uncommon anemia caused by the breakdown of circulating red blood cells.
- Invasion of the bone marrow by cancer, leukemia, or multiple myeloma causes anemia as normal red blood cells are crowded out by neoplastic disease.

Other diseases that may lead to anemia include chronic infection, hypersplenism, drug sensitivity, regional enteritis, and any of a dozen more.

This plethora of possible causes of anemia is presented not as a guide to home diagnosis, but to emphasize the many diagnostic possibilities when anemia is encountered. Remember: Unless the cause of anemia is obvious (for example, a tea-and-toast diet), it's a diagnostic problem that calls for the doctor's best detective efforts.

ANGINA

Synonym: angina pectoris

The pressure pain of angina pectoris is caused by a shortage of blood to the heart. Heart muscles depends upon oxygen carried to it by tiny arteries, and when arteriosclerosis (see Atherosclerosis) or cholesterol plaques partially block the arterial passageways, the heart muscle receives a marginal blood supply. All may be well until the heart is called upon for extra effort, such as pushing a car, responding to a crisis, or combating illness. Then the heart's blood supply fails to satisfy its need, and the heart muscle cries plaintively in pain.

The symptoms of angina pectoris were described, and indeed first named, in the following paragraphs from *Com-*

mentaries on the History and Cure of Diseases by William Heberden in the eighteenth century:

> There is a disorder of the breast marked with strong and peculiar symptoms, considerable for the kind of danger belonging to it, and not extremely rare, which deserves to be mentioned more at length. The seat of it, and sense of strangling and anxiety with which it is attended, may make it not improperly be called angina pectoris. They who are afflicted with it, are seized while they are walking (more especially if it be uphill, and soon after eating) with a painful and most disagreeable sensation in the breast, which seems as if it would extinguish life, if it were to increase or to continue; but the moment they stand still, all this uneasiness vanished.

Doctor Heberden touched upon the four critical factors in angina pectoris. First, it begins with a disagreeable sensation in the chest, usually described as oppressive in nature, as though the ribs and breast bone are being squeezed tightly, and often traveling to the shoulder, arm, or jaw (see Figure 2). Walking uphill may be the precipitating factor, or it may follow snow shoveling, the first tennis game in ten years, or other unaccustomed exertion.

Anxiety plays a role, and angina is an ever-present threat to the tension-ridden executive. Fourth, while angina may not always vanish upon standing still, rest reduces the heart's need for oxygen-carrying blood and shortens the duration of an acute anginal attack.

Patients often ask? "What's the difference between angina pectoris and a heart attack?"

Here's the answer: Both result from atherosclerosis (*q.v.*) of the blood vessels leading to the heart, and both are likely to follow some combination of anxiety, overeating, vigorous physical exertion, and perhaps exposure to cold weather. Furthermore, both angina and a heart attack are characterized by a pressure-type severe mid-chest pain often radiating to the shoulders, arm, or jaw, and sometimes attended by shortness of breath.

But here's the difference: Angina pectoris, by definition, is a temporary shortage of blood to the heart. It is brief and reversible, causing no permanent damage.

A heart attack, on the other hand, results in some per-

15

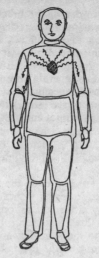

FIGURE 2. *Radiation of anginal pain.*

manent damage to the heart muscle. The supply of life-sustaining blood falls and that portion of heart muscle supplied by the tiny blocked artery dies—to soften and subsequently to be replaced by scar tissue over the following weeks.

Angina pectoris may be, and often is, the forerunner of a heart attack. And yet I know one individual who suffered anginal attacks almost daily for twenty years until he died at age eighty-five of causes unrelated to his heart.

On the brighter side, the pain of angina may be taken as a warning, alerting the self-helper to the need for a reduced load on his heart.

The Role of Self-Help Treatment

Mention angina and most folks think: nitroglycerin. But there's much that self-help therapy can do to supplement medication prescribed by the doctor.

First, stop smoking! Cigarettes are the most hazardous, but the inhalation of pipe and cigar smoke also takes its toll in angina pectoris. To tip the odds in your favor, smoking must cease.

Trim excess weight. Every pound of fat adds almost a mile of tiny capillaries through which the heart must pump blood. Eliminating needless extra weight reduces the strain on the heart and lowers the likelihood that angina will strike.

While eliminating excess calories from the diet, try to trim dietary cholesterol and fats. Cholesterol and lipids accelerate atherosclerosis, and fats provide more than their share of calories. Unless a more specific diet is prescribed by the physician after lipid analysis (see Atherosclerosis), the following is a useful diet low in fat and cholesterol.

Low Cholesterol, Low Fat Diet

Foods Permitted	*Foods to Be Avoided*
Cereals	
Cooked oat and wheat cereals	Sugar-coated cereals
Dry precooked cereals	
Bran cereals	
Breads	
2 slices of white bread or whole wheat bread	Muffins, rolls, and biscuits
	Corn bread
	Pancakes and waffles
Soups	
Bouillon and broth	Creamed soups
	Meat-stock soups
	Bean, lentil, or split pea
Meat, Fish, and Dairy Products	
Boiled, baked, or broiled veal, ham, lean beef turkey or chicken, and fish	Mutton and pork
	Fried or fatty meats
	Shellfish
Cottage cheese (preferably uncreamed)	Soft cooked eggs
	Fried eggs
	Cheese, except cottage cheese
Vegetables	
All raw and cooked vegetables	
Fruits	
All raw and cooked fruits	
Fruit juices	

Foods Permitted	Foods to Be Avoided

Desserts

Sherbet	Cakes
Gelatin	Pies and pastries
Bread pudding } made with	Custard and puddings
Rice pudding } skimmed milk	Ice cream

Beverages

Decaffeinated coffee	Coffee, tea, and alcohol
Cocoa, Postum, and Ovaltine	Carbonated beverages
Skimmed milk	Whole milk
	Buttermilk

Miscellaneous

Liquid vegetable oils (corn, soybean, and safflower oils)	Animal fats and lard
	Olives
Pepper	Salt
Pickles	Mayonnaise
Macaroni and spaghetti	Gravy
Tomato paste	Salted and unsalted nuts
Garlic	Sugar and candy
Mustard	
Horseradish	
Jelly and jam	
Relish	
Vinegar	

Avoid stress that might bring on an acute attack of angina. Each individual is likely to have one or two factors to which he is particularly susceptible. I know one executive who can play handball all afternoon, yet suffers angina while debating at board meetings. A truck driver patient of mine has described how he can work an 18-hour day, contend with on-the-job aggravation, yet suffers angina when he leaves the house each morning if the temperature is below 20 degrees. Other individuals suffer angina only when precipitating causes occur in combination, such as during a brisk walk after a big meal. Below is a list of factors that, singly or in combination, may induce an acute attack in the angina-prone individual:

- Overeating, particularly the feasts likely to accompany the Thanksgiving or Christmas holidays.
- Unaccustomed physical exertion, such as pushing a car or shoveling winter snow.

- Acute and chronic aggravation, nagging frustration at work, or an acute anxiety-producing situation such as death of a loved one, divorce, or a big financial deal gone sour.
- Extremely cold weather, especially when the "I don't get sick" he-man goes outdoors without proper winter clothing.

Gradually increasing exercise can boost the heart's tolerance. Of course it's all-important to begin very gradually, and this can't be overemphasized in self-help of the anginal syndrome. Doctor James I. Thompson of Duluth, Minnesota recommends walking, jogging, running, stationary bicycling, and swimming, but discourages isometric exercises, which place an undue strain on the heart.

Start by walking—two or three times each day, preferably when the stomach is not overfull, and not during blustery winter weather. Lengthen the route a little each day, gradually increasing the pace. After a few months, you've become a brisk walker and, if your physician gives his okay, may even jog a few steps from time to time. Once stamina has been increased, ask your physician for his prescription for a graded conditioning program—such as the one described in *Adult Physical Fitness—A Program for Men and Women* (published by The President's Council on Physical Fitness, available from the Superintendent of Documents, U.S. Government Printing Office, Washington, D.C. 20402, 35 cents).

Always keep in mind that graded exercise can increase the heart's endurance, while sudden bursts of frantic physical activity can place that organ in peril.

Don't stop here. The anginal syndrome demands expert medical evaluation—and follow-up. Consult your physician.

What the Doctor Can Do for Angina

Aside from advice concerning weight control, dietary fats and cholesterol, habits, and exercise, the doctor has at his disposal three general types of drugs to help angina:

- Nitroglycerin, available in 0.3 and 0.4-mg tablets, is taken under the tongue to quickly abort an anginal attack. Effective within two minutes if it is going to work at all, nitroglycerin should be taken as early as possible during the anginal attack. In fact, some individuals take nitroglycerin tablets sublingually (under the tongue) in anticipation of angina—just before performing an activity (such as opening the garage door on a frosty morning or just prior to sexual relations) to prevent the angina that otherwise might occur.

- The long-acting coronary vasodilators are medications taken two, three, or four times daily to help prevent attacks of angina. The great granddaddy of such medication is pentaerythritol tetranitrate (Peritrate), and it remains a standard in the field. Other available medications include erythrityl tetranitrate (Cardilate), isosorbide dinitrate (Isordil), or timed-release nitroglycerin (Nitro-Bid).

- Propranolol hydrochloride (Inderal) stands in a class by itself. Newest of the antianginal agents, propranolol reduces the heart's need for oxygen, thus reducing anginal attacks. The dosage varies from 10 to 80 mg three or four times daily and has been, in my experience, a most useful drug in controling angina pectoris.

Besides securing his advice and prescription for medication, there's one further reason for contacting the physician. If angina should fail to subside within 30 to 60 minutes, perhaps after taking three or four nitroglycerin pills, the physician should be called; a heart attack (see page 150) may have occurred. At this time, it's most helpful to be able to call a doctor who has prior knowledge (and perhaps past electrocardiograms) of your cardiac status.

ANIMAL BITE

Any youngster can be nipped by a passing dog, bitten by a not-so-tame squirrel, or gashed while trying to help a wounded woodland animal. Whatever the bite, basic principles apply, requiring attention to local therapy, tetanus prophylaxis, and the possibility of rabies.

Local Treatment

Examine the wound, questioning to be sure the injury is a bite and not just a scratch from the animal's nail (in which case rabies would not be a source of worry). Remove all clothing from the local area and scrub thoroughly with water and soap—Ivory Soap is fine, pHisoHex (available by prescription only) is better. Then rinse thoroughly with plenty of water, allow to dry in the air, and apply povidone-iodine (Betadine) solution. Cover with a sterile gauze bandage. Then call the doctor if a gaping wound may need stitches or if tetanus and/or rabies prophylaxis is in question.

Tetanus Prevention

The bite of any animal may cause tetanus, particularly if there is a puncture wound that could deposit germs deep beneath the skin. Careful cleansing helps, perhaps followed by warm saline soaks three times daily at home. But the most reliable tetanus prophylaxis is the booster shot, and if the bitten individual hasn't had a tetanus booster within a year or two, the doctor should be contacted for his advice.

Preventing Rabies

What to do about rabies takes judgment. Each year there are more than two million animal bites resulting in more than 30,000 courses of rabies shots, and only one or two Americans develop rabies. Yet the astronomical mortality of human rabies, the uncertain health of the biting animal, the formidable complications of rabies vaccine administration, and the prospect of 14 to 21 painful daily injections all pose a ponderous dilemma to the parents and doctor of a child bitten by a strange animal.

The type of bite is considered. Most likely to harbor rabies are carnivorous animals: foxes, raccoons, coyotes, skunks, dogs, and cats. Rodent herbivores are much less likely to be rabid; bites of squirrels, mice, hamsters, and even rats seldom require antirabies vaccines.

How did the bite occur? Was a youngster nipped while trying to separate two quarreling housecats? Little chance of rabies here. Or was the child a victim of an unprovoked attack by a wandering dog or woodland animal?

In general, antirabies vaccine is recommended for individuals suffering severe bites from an animal with signs suggestive of rabies or if the animal is unknown and escapes capture. Bites of known rabid animals or those of a skunk, coyote, raccoon, fox, or bat that attack without provocation are considered potentially rabid and vaccine is begun immediately. In the end, the decision to give or withhold rabies vaccine is made jointly by the physician and patient (or parents), based upon consideration of all factors involved.

ANKLE SPRAIN

The sprained ankle can be treacherous. An inward twisting of the ankle stretches and often tears vital ligaments, and may mask a broken bone. Swelling is noted and the area is warm to the touch. There is pain upon walking and, if a small blood vessel has broken, a large black-and-blue patch may be present. The area is sore to the touch, particularly the soft spot below the bony prominence on the outside of the ankle; tenderness of the bone above this point suggests a fracture.

Nevertheless, none of these signs can reliably distinguish between a sprained ankle and a fracture, and an x-ray should be taken.

Treatment

Mild ankle sprains are treated with rest, support, and moist compresses. Rest means not walking on the involved extremity, and crutches may be necessary. A three-inch Ace Bandage applied in a figure-of-eight fashion lends support; remove and reapply the elastic bandage several times daily, not too tightly, and remove the support at bedtime.

The ankle sprain, like other acute soft-tissue injuries, is treated with compresses as follows: Cold applications are applied intermittently during the first 24 hours to reduce swelling. After the first day, warm, moist applications bring blood into the area and promote healing.

If the sprain has been mild, limited weight-bearing is possible after four to seven days, but full activity should not be resumed for several weeks and active sports should be deferred for one to two months.

ANXIETY

Synonyms: nervousness, anxiety neurosis

With prices bounding ever upward; the constant threat of shortages of fuel, food, and who-knows-what next year; and the ever-present possibility that some misguided political leader may trigger a nuclear holocaust, it's scant wonder that many individuals suffer anxiety.

Anxiety—it's the burst of speed that helped the caveman escape the sabre-toothed tiger; it's the stomach queasiness the actor feels on opening night; it's the trembling following a near-accident in your car. When it occurs in times of stress, anxiety helps us cope, but nervousness can be troublesome when it lasts all day long.

The symptoms of anxiety are varied: sometimes a mild tremor of the hands, often sweaty palms, perhaps there is stammering speech, rapid blinking is frequently noted, and there may be headaches, indigestion, or diarrhea. A common outlet for nervous tension is hyperventilation—an anxious compulsion to take deep sighing breaths.

Whatever the outward manifestations, most anxious individuals share an ever-present, overpowering sense of impending doom, as if spending their lives teetering on the brink of a disaster they can't describe.

Alleviating Anxiety

Self-help medical therapy of anxiety begins by examining the cause. It won't be easy. The sources of anxiety are seldom obvious and are often deeply rooted in the subconscious. Yet the search is worth the effort because once the origins of anxiety are uncovered, the battle is half won. Conflicts are defined and decisions made; that's the key to resolving most situation-induced anxiety. The college graduate vacillates between professional school and a job offer; the middle-ager is torn between his sense of responsibility and the urge to chuck it all; the oldster ponders whether he should keep up the family home or move to a retirement village. The fact of making a decision, whether or not it later turns out to be "right," does much to allay anxiety.

Of course, there's more—the minute-by-minute, hour-by-hour assault on equanimity: the fourth telephone call in fifteen minutes, the noise of jets overhead, children fighting over an object they'll both ignore ten minutes later, repairmen that don't show up. Anxiety-charged situations should be avoided whenever possible. That means dodging downtown traffic, even if you must drive an extra ten minutes on quiet country roads. It means shopping when the stores aren't crowded, even if you must arise an hour earlier in the morning. And it means reducing responsibilities that often beget anxiety, even if you must decline a coveted promotion or reject a prestigious chairmanship.

Always keep in mind that anxiety is a symptom, not a disease in itself. It's a reaction to a mental conflict—with the body churning out adrenalin to meet the crisis. Resolve or avoid the conflict, and anxiety is lessened.

If anxiety is your nemesis, learn all you can about the disorder. There's a wealth of information available, and good sources of literature are:

American Mental Health Foundation
2 East 86th Street
New York, New York 10028

The National Association for Mental Health, Inc.
10 Columbus Circle
New York, New York 10019

Drug Treatment

Several over-the-counter preparations are earmarked for anxiety. Their effect comes from antihistamines—usually pyrilamine or methapyrilene—also sometimes used as mild sleeping pills. A few over-the-counter sedatives also contain scopolamine (a derivative of belladonna) or caffeine. Cope Tablets contain methapyrilene fumarate, aspirin, and caffeine with aluminum magnesium (I wonder if the caffeine may not offset methapyrilene's tranquilizing properties). In Compoz Tablets we find methapyrilene hydrochloride, pyrilamine maleate, and a small dose of scopolamine. This seems to me a more rational formula, eliminating aspirin that may cause stomach irritation and potentially stimulating caffeine.

Other no-prescription-needed sedatives containing antihistamines are available, including Sleep-eze Tablets, Sominex Tablets, and Nytol Tablets and Capsules—all containing relatively larger doses of methapyrilene and widely advertised as sleeping pills.

The use of over-the-counter sedatives is a short-term crutch, helping combat temporary anxiety until emotional conflicts are resolved. In many instances, the very fact of taking medication is reassuring, and I wonder if the chief benefit of many over-the-counter and prescription sedatives does not derive from their placebo value.

When to Call the Doctor

Sometimes anxiety overwhelms, self-help analysis fizzles, and nonprescription sedatives just won't do the job. Then it's time for professional counseling, and perhaps a prescription tranquilizer to soothe jangled nerves.

Professional counseling helps exorcise the anxiety neurosis—aiding your analysis of conflict and helping to reach important decisions. Turn to your family physician first, although the busy forty-patient-a-day practitioner will often refer you to a counselor. A psychiatrist isn't always needed and, in fact, most individuals receiving counseling are treated by psychotherapists—trained clinical psychologists who help them work out their problems. Your family physician, usually on a first-name basis with counselors in the local areas, may make the referral. Or you may prefer to send a note to the American Psychiatric Association, 1700 Eighteenth Street, NW., Washington, D.C. 20009, or the American Psychological Association, 1200 Seventeenth Street, N.W., Washington, D.C. 20036; ask for the names of therapists in your local area.

The family physician or psychotherapist will often prescribe an antianxiety agent. Common choices are chlordiazepoxide (Librium), diazepam (Valium), oxazapam (Serax) or meprobamate (Equanil). These mild tranquilizers help alleviate symptoms until anxiety-producing conflicts are resolved. Look upon them as you would taking aspirin for a headache; it relieves symptoms, but does not really attack the cause.

Yes, there's much that can be done when anxiety strikes. Self-analysis is worth a try, perhaps supplemented by over-the-counter medication, but severe anxiety should not be long endured before seeking medical help and, perhaps, professional counseling.

APHTHOUS ULCER

Synonym: canker sore

As its victims will tell you, the aphthous ulcer is more painful than it looks. There's a gray-white erosion of the skin, surrounded by a red halo, usually found in the valley between the cheeks and gums. Some individuals say aphthous ulcers are due to emotional turmoil, others blame the monthly menstrual period, while still others relate them to citrus fruit, sugar, or other foods.

In fact, the cause is unknown, although many doctors insist they're a type of virus infection.

Treatment

Avoiding known causative foods helps, and we should all try to sidestep contagious disease and needless emotional stress. Nevertheless, aphthous ulcers frequently occur. The following list of possible treatments is testimony that no one of them is dramatically effective:

- Gly-oxide Liquid containing carbamide peroxide has been my favorite anti-canker sore preparation. It's applied undiluted to the sore four times daily, either with a swab or directly from the squeeze bottle. Contact is maintained for two to three minutes, followed by expectoration.
- Benzodent Ointment, an anesthetic preparation for use on gums, may bring transient relief.
- Triamcinolone Acetonide 0.1 percent (Kenalog) in Orabase may be prescribed by the doctor.
- Doctor Robert Webster of Atlanta, Georgia recommends application of a moist teabag. Dip the teabag in boiling water, squeeze out most of the water. Allow it to cool slightly, then apply to the canker sore for two to three minutes. The active ingredient is probably tannic acid, and pressure with the moist teabag

26

has also been used to stop bleeding from a tooth socket after extraction.

- In Fresno, California, Dr. B. Peck Lau advises pressing a wetted aspirin tablet against the aphthous ulcer until the initial stinging has subsided. Follow by rinsing the mouth five minutes later, and a thin whitish film will be left that crusts over in about 24 hours.

- Warm saline gargles with one-half teaspoonful of table salt dissolved in eight ounces of fairly hot water, swirled in the mouth and expectorated until the entire eight ounces has been used. Try it in conjunction with whatever other therapy is tried. It can't hurt and it's free.

APPENDICITIS

Self-help treatment of appendicitis has just one goal: bringing to mind the correct diagnosis so the patient receives surgery promptly. To this end, let's review the textbook symptoms and signs of acute appendicitis.

The patient is usually a youngster, teen-ager, or young adult, and symptoms will be of relatively short duration. The pain begins as a vague discomfort in the upper abdomen or around the navel and at first is crampy in nature. Slight nausea is present, there may be an episode of vomiting and/or a few loose bowel movements. A low-grade fever is not uncommon, but temperatures exceeding 102°F. are usually not caused by appendicitis. The patient characteristically loses his appetite, and I put great stock in the old adage that the individual with appendicitis did not eat his last meal.

Within a few hours, the pain moves to the right lower quadrant of the abdomen (see Figure 3)—the area where the appendix is located. Also there's a change in the nature of the pain, which becomes more intense and constant than before. Walking may induce pain, and the individual riding in a car feels acute discomfort when the car bounces.

A light touch on the abdomen, particularly over the right lower quadrant site of pain brings a cry of protest.

When the patient's symptoms fit this pattern, call the doctor without delay—even if it's two o'clock in the morning. Immediate evaluation is mandatory, and if appendicitis is present, surgery within a few hours is needed to prevent perforation. Under no circumstances should a laxative be administered, a heating pad be applied to the abdomen, or other temporizing maneuvers be allowed to consume precious time that should be spent seeking medical advice.

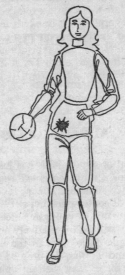

FIGURE 3. *Usual site of appendicitis pain.*

When Appendicitis Doesn't Follow the Book

If only diseases came with handy labels and the appendicitis victim could be counted upon to match the textbook description! But it's not to be, and appendicitis can be fickle as a courtesan. Sometimes the disease attacks infants, usually resulting in perforation before the diagnosis is made. Other times oldsters are afflicted, and gallstones or peptic ulcer disease may be suspected—almost anything but appendicitis. In other instances the victim is the "right" age, but the pain is in the wrong place, perhaps due to an inflamed appendix tucked down behind the large intestine. Still other diseased appendixes mimic ovulation pain, menstrual cramps, or even acute constipation.

Why tell all this? It's to emphasize that abdominal pain, particularly in a young individual (who still has his appendix) should never be neglected. As a practicing physician, I'll always jump from bed to check out this complaint, because I know that any individual with abdominal pain just might have an acute appendicitis.

ARTHRITIS

Synonym: rheumatism

Arthritis is a catchall term describing a mixed bag of joint diseases, the common denominator being inflammation of one or more joints. At least 14 million Americans have arthritis in one form or another, including five million individuals with potentially crippling rheumatoid arthritis. The economic impact of arthritis is staggering, with an estimated annual wage loss of up to $2 billion due to the disease, not to mention several hundred million dollars spent for remedies of dubious value.

By far the most common type of arthritis is osteoarthritis, also called degenerative arthritis, a disease of aging as wear and tear grinds down the protective cartilage at bone ends. A painful grating sensation at the joints may be accompanied by bone spurs. Often involved are weight-bearing joints, especially the knees, and a characteristic deformity is a knobby enlargement of the last joint of the fingers called Heberden's nodes (see Figure 4). Joint pain is the chief complaint, aggravated by activity and changing weather conditions. Some might argue that osteoarthritis is a physiologic consequence of aging, but the discomfort in joints that it causes more than justifies its inclusion as an arthritic disease.

Rheumatoid arthritis is a horse of a different color, striking young adults in the prime of life, causing hot, swollen, painful joints, and often culminating in deformity. Ralph Waldo Emerson wrote of "writhing and roaring in our beds with rheumatism," highlighting the extreme discomfort and debility that can attend rheumatoid arthritis. In time, chronic joint inflammation can cause a shifting of bones within joints, often involving the fingers and knees, severely hampering the use of these joints and earning for the disease the medical name arthritis deformans.

Even before consulting the physician, there's much that can be done to fight arthritis of both types, including easing the stress placed upon joints, physical therapy, and use of nonprescription analgesics.

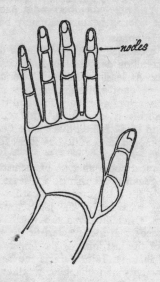

FIGURE 4. *Heberden's nodes of osteoarthritis.*

Protecting joints from needless strain is a good starting point. Weight reduction relieves the burden that must be borne by joints of the spine, hips, knees, and ankles; the overweight arthritic should undertake a calorie control program (see Obesity) aimed at attaining his ideal weight.

Sometimes arthritis follows repetitive use (or abuse) of a joint. For example, a middle-aged woman may develop arthritis of her shoulder after many years of tugging at a clothesline pulley. When arthritic pains are related to a specific activity, it's time to look for another way to get that particular job done.

Heat helps most arthritic joints feel better. Moist heat penetrates better than dry, and hot packs with a damp towel, or a hot bath, will usually be superior to a plain heating pad application. A useful device that can be purchased with prescription is the Hydrocollator Pad, an absorbent pad designed to hold heat and moisture against the skin. During acute flare-ups moist heat is applied to a painful joint for 30 to 60 minutes four times daily. Be wary of burns, possible with any type of heat, but particularly likely to occur with heating pad overuse. (Remember, moist packs will cool with time, while the electric heating pad may become hotter and hotter.)

Exercise helps prevent joint stiffness. Each joint has a certain range of motion. Try it. The elbow, a hinge joint, will flex and extend, while the ball-and-socket shoulder joint can move up, forward, back, and down. While overuse should be avoided, an arthritic joint should be moved through its full range of motion two or three times daily to preserve mobility and to prevent unnecessary stiffening.

Diet therapy of arthritis enjoys an occasional flurry of publicity, yet no specific diet has ever been found to alleviate joint disease. Fad diets should be avoided, and the following basic nutritional guidelines should be observed:

- Take adequate protein to allow repair of damaged joints.
- If undernutrition is suspected, assure that adequate calories are consumed.
- When weight reduction is necessary, trim high-calorie carbohydrates and fats in the diet.
- Take one or two servings of calcium-containing milk products daily to allow bone repair.
- Take a multivitamin supplement such as Optilet-M-500 Vitamins daily.
- One old-fashioned remedy for arthritis is parsley, and grandma's recipe is as follows: Boil a handful of parsley (stems included) in a pint of water, left to simmer for 30 minutes. The full pint should be consumed as three or more large cups of tea each day.

Nonprescription drug treatment refers to the use of aspirin and its cousin acetaminophen. Aspirin (acetylsalicylic acid) has been in use since 1899 and remains a standard in the treatment of arthritis. For severe arthritis, aspirin is often taken in doses of eight tablets daily, sometimes more. Because high dosages can cause stomach irritation and sometimes bleeding, it is often advisable to pay the few extra cents for aspirin with aluminum-magnesium buffers (Bufferin), aspirin with a film coating to prevent disintegration in the stomach (Ecotrin), aspirin with Maalox brand of magnesium-aluminum hydroxide (Ascriptin), or liquid choline salicylate (Arthropan). When taking relatively large doses of aspirin over a prolonged period of time, it also helps to consume the medication with meals or perhaps with a glass of milk.

Acetaminophen (Tylenol) is less likely than aspirin to irritate the stomach lining and has been used by many arthritics who cannot tolerate aspirin-containing products. Although some physicians would disagree, Dr. David S. Howell, writing in *Conn's Current Therapy*, states, "Acetaminophen (Tylenol) is often as effective, in my opinion, as equal doses of aspirin."

How about the welter of pain-killers available on drugstore shelves? Pay the price for brand name advertising if you please, but be sure to read the label and know what you are taking. For example, Anacin merely contains aspirin and caffeine; aspirin is much less expensive when purchased generically, while caffeine is of doubtful value in arthritis and may cause a jittery nervous feeling. Empirin compound contains phenacetin (whose excessive use can cause kidney damage), aspirin, and caffeine. Widely advertised Excedrin combines small doses of acetaminophen, aspirin, caffeine, and salicylamide (another of the aspirin family). Nebs and Valadol each contain 325 mg (five grains) of acetaminophen, while Measurin contains 10 grains of time-release aspirin.

Whether the disease is rheumatoid or osteoarthritis, over-the-counter analgesics can be helpful. Choose wisely, keeping in mind that the most useful ingredients are aspirin and acetaminophen, that the manufacturer's recommendations must be followed carefully, and that the drug should be stopped promptly if side effects occur.

The Doctor and Arthritis

The physician has much to offer the arthritic, and self-help medical care should supplement, but not replace, professional guidance. Of paramount importance is the precise diagnosis, requiring a physical examination by the physician, perhaps aided by blood tests and x-rays. What seems to be rheumatoid or osteoarthritis may turn out to be gout (*q.v.*), a joint infection, or any of several other joint disorders.

Once the diagnosis is established, the physician can offer guidance concerning home treatment, including applications of heat, range-of-motion exercises, isometric exercises, and diet. He may prescribe an orthopedic appliance or support such as a hinged knee brace, a wrist support with velcro attachment, or a sling to rest an aching shoulder joint.

Prescription drug treatment is recommended when simple measures don't do the job. One or more of the following drugs may be prescribed, often taken in conjunction with aspirin or acetaminophen:

- Propoxyphene (Darvon) is a painkiller available in a host of dosage forms, including combinations with aspirin and acetaminophen. It probably has little or no advantage over aspirin and, like others in this list, can cause stomach irritation.

- Indomethacin (Indocin) gets to the heart of joint inflammation and has been a useful drug in most forms of arthritis. Three or four 25-mg capsules is the usual starting dose, best taken with meals. Stomach irritation, lightheadedness, and headaches are the possible side effects, and indomethacin can stir up a previously quiet peptic ulcer.

- Ibuprofen (Motrin) made its American debut in 1974 and has since proved its worth as a safe and effective antiarthritis remedy. The dose is one 400-mg tablet four times daily and Motrin can often be used by individuals whose stomachs won't tolerate aspirin or Indocin.

- Naproxen (Naprosyn) and Tolmetin (Tolectin), recently approved by the FDA for the treatment of arthritis, seem to have actions and side effects similar to ibuprofen.

- Phenylbutazone (Butazoladin) is another antiinflammatory agent taken three or four times daily with meals. The response to phenylbutazone is usually prompt and therapy with this drug is usually of brief duration, owing to its formidable possible side effects—stomach irritation, bleeding ulcers, fluid retention, and anemia.

- Cortisone tablets, prescribed more often for rheumatoid arthritis than for osteoarthritis, provide dramatic improvement but are also best taken for only a few weeks at a time. Prolonged use can cause fluid retention, bleeding ulcers, softening of the bones, diabetes, and more. Sometimes cortisone compounds such as Aristocort or Depo-Medrol are given by direct injection into the joint, perhaps mixed with pain-killing lidocaine (Xylocaine).

- Gold injections (Solganal or Myocrysine) are sometimes recommended for severe rheumatoid arthritis unresponsive to less potent measures; gold is not useful in the treatment of osteoarthritis or other joint diseases. Available only by injection, gold is given in a series of weekly shots, with careful monitoring for the side effects of itching, skin rash, and sore mouth. Gold's usefulness is limited by the inconvenience of frequent injections, its cost, and its potential hazards, yet of the many drugs to treat arthritis, only gold and aspirin have track records of more than thirty years of use.

- Antimalarials such as chloroquine (Aralen) and hydroxychloroquine (Plaquenil) are occasionally prescribed for severe rheumatoid arthritis. The doctor must balance the possible benefits of an antimalarial against its possible hazards, including anemia, skin rash, and damage to the retina of the eye, and on balance he usually decides against its use.

Reconstructive surgery is sometimes recommended for advanced arthritis, particularly for joints that have become severely deformed, unstable, excessively stiffened, or whose function can otherwise by improved surgically. Possible operations include removal of a painfully overgrown joint lining, removal of loose bodies within knee joints, fusion of a severely arthritic thumb joint, relief of pressure on the nerve at the wrist, or even total replacement of the hip or knee joint. Further advice and help for the arthritic is available from:

The Arthritis Foundation
1212 Avenue of the Americas

New York, New York 10036
(Ask for the booklet *Strike Back at Arthritis*.)

National Institute of Arthritis and Metabolic Diseases
Room 9AOA, Building 31
National Institute of Health
Bethesda, Maryland 20014

Merck, Sharp & Dohme, makers of Indocin, publish a
Helpful Booklet for the Patient with Arthritis, describing diet,
exercises, and ways that household chores can be made easier
for the arthritic. It is available from your physician or by
writing:

Merck, Sharp & Dohme
West Point, Pennsylvania 19486

ASBESTOSIS

Here's all the information I can offer the self-help medical
practitioner about asbestosis: It's a chronic lung disease
caused by inhalation of asbestos particles, usually following
many years of occupational exposure. It causes shortness of
breath, progressive if exposure continues. The only treatment
available is simple: Cease all inhalation of asbestos particles.

ASTHMA

Synonym: bronchial asthma

The asthmatic fights to breathe, and all his efforts are consumed in moving air into and out of the lungs. The victim
sits quietly, often with forearms braced on the table so that
he can use his shoulder and chest muscles to breathe. He
talks little, saving his breath, and the loudest sound may be a
wheeze during expiration.

Bronchial asthma is related to allergy, and may occur
when pollen levels are high. Atmospheric conditions play a
role, and asthma attacks may occur during periods of chang-

ing weather. In other individuals, the wheezing of asthma begins following emotional upheaval or exposure to irritating fumes.

Self-help treatment of asthma includes preventing and relieving acute attacks, although severe episodes of wheezing are best managed by the physician.

Preventing Asthma Attacks

The asthmatic soon learns that he can't tolerate smoke-filled rooms. Allergy-producing substances are also best avoided, including pollens, house dust, and animal dander. Sometimes this means banishing a household pet or parting with a down-stuffed sofa, but the alleviation of asthma can be dramatic when an allergenic is eliminated.

Preventing colds and other infections can help sidestep asthmatic wheezing. This means avoiding crowds, dressing properly when going outdoors, eating nutritious meals with plenty of vitamins, and getting a full quota of sleep.

Some individuals find that a small dose of an expectorant, such as glyceryl guaiacolate (Robitussin), taken as one teaspoonful three or four times daily, helps keep bronchial passages clear and minimizes asthma attacks.

Other persons prevent asthma attacks by sporadic use of capsules or tablets to keep the bronchi open. Top-notch over-the-counter preparations are;

- Asthmanefrin Capsules containing pseudoephedrine, theophylline, methapyrilene hydrochloride and glyceryl guaiacolate.
- Bronkotabs, containing ephedrine sulfate, theophylline, phenyldiamine hydrochloride, phenobarbital, and glyceryl guaiacolate.
- Tedral Tablets, containing ephedrine hydrochloride, theophylline, and phenobarbital.

Relieving the Acute Asthma Attack

When an acute episode of wheezing occurs, urgent treatment is needed. First may come a double dose of Asthmanefrin, Bronkotabs, or Tedral Tablets this will help open tightened bronchial tubes.

Thick dried-out secretions hamper breathing in asthma, and I encourage patients to drink water, one glass after another, while other medicine is being administered. Even if vomiting ensues, it helps clear secretions from the chest.

Inhalers can bring speedy relief in acute asthma, thanks to the bronchial-opening properties of epinephrine. Available without prescription is Bronkaid Aerosol Mist or Primatene Aerosol Mist, one spray of each delivering about 0.2 mg of epinephrine by inhalation. Epinephrine inhalers are potent and should be treated with respect; too many whiffs can cause a rapid heartbeat and bounding blood pressure, while chronic overuse can bring a psychological (and to some degree, physical) dependence, along with resistance to epinephrine by injection.

If these measures fail, call the doctor immediately.

What the Physician Has to Offer

Relieving the acute asthma attack is one of the doctor's most satisfying challenges. A patient in severe respiratory distress often can be relieved within minutes, thanks to the doctor's skillful injection of epinephrine, cortisone, or perhaps aminophylline. Occasionally several shots are needed, and every so often hospitalization is recommended for prolonged treatment.

Once the acute episode is over, the physician may prescribe cromolyn sodium (Aarane) to inhibit the release of asthma-stimulating histamine and help prevent future attacks. Or perhaps he will suggest allergy testing and densensitization shots in an effort to abolish recurrent bouts of asthma.

ATHEROSCLEROSIS

Synonyms: arteriosclerosis, hardening of the arteries

Atherosclerosis is a prime public health problem, and its complications—heart disease, stroke, and hypertension—are the leading causes of death in the United States today. Autopsies performed on servicemen during the Korean War revealed that young Americans had a startling incidence of atherosclerosis when compared with their Oriental counterparts. The cause? Many factors contribute, including diet, exercise, heredity, and other influences that science has yet to discover.

Attacking Atherosclerosis

The prevention of atherosclerosis and its consequences should begin during childhood, although it's probably never too late to start. Here's a self-help plan to allay atherosclerosis:

- Cut calories, to attain and hold your ideal body weight. This means eliminating empty calories found in sweets and soft drinks, substituting nutritious fruits, vegetables, and low-fat meats. Eliminating excess adiposity shortens the miles of capillaries through which the heart must pump blood, lowering the blood pressure and relieving the strain on vital arteries.
- Exercise regularly, including conditioning (aerobic) exercises such as jogging and/or swimming to stimulate circulation and improve muscle tone. If your last exercise session was a high school gym class, begin slowly. A few sit-ups and stretching exercises will do for the first day, adding a few repetitions and perhaps a new drill every few days. It's much more beneficial to exercise for 10 minutes daily than to expend a burst of frantic activity just once a week. Figure 5 illustrates a training program for home use by Professor Per-Olof Åstrand, M.D., of the Gymnastik och Idrottshögskolan, Stockholm, Sweden, and reprinted here with the permission Skandia Insurance Company Ltd. of Stockholm and the President's Council on Physical Fitness.
- Learn to relax, including daily periods of physical and emotional rest, and frequent short vacations. A quiet lunch, a few minutes alone at day's end, the cup of coffee by the fireplace in the evening—they are all ways to balance the tension of the day's duties. A once-a-year three-week vacation is fine, but many busy individuals find it's more relaxing to take a long weekend each month, or perhaps a few one-week vacations each year. It's well known that a prolonged period of hectic activity can precede a heart attack,

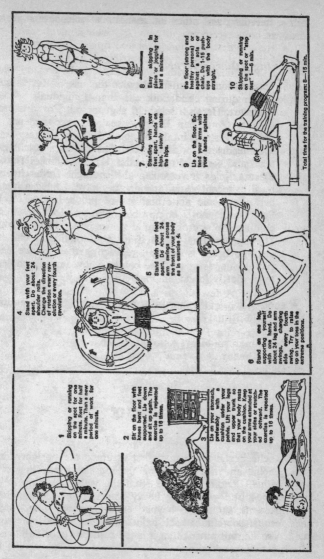

Total time for the training program: 8—15 min.

8 Easy skipping in place or jogging for half a minute.

7 Standing with your feet apart, hands on hips, slowly rotate the hips.

the floor (strong and healthy persons) or against a sofa or chair. Do 1-15 push-ups with the body straight.

9 Lie on the floor. Extend your arms with your hands against

10 Skipping or running on the spot or "spot test" 1—5 min.

4 Stand with your feet apart. Do about 24 shoulder rolls. Change the direction of rotation every fourth revolution or every fourth revolution.

5 Stand with your feet apart. Do about 24 arm swings across the front of your body as in exercise 4.

6 Stand on one leg, supporting yourself with one hand. Do about 24 leg and arm swings, changing sides every fourth swing. Try to raise up your toes in the extreme positions.

1 Skipping or running on the spot for one minute. Rest for half a minute. Then a new period of work for one minute.

2 Sit on the floor with knees bent and feet supported. Lie down and sit up. The exercise is repeated up to 10 times.

3 Lie on your stomach, preferably with a cushion under your pelvis. Lift your legs and upper trunk so that your body rests on the cushion. Keep your arms extended at your sides and stretched outward. The exercise is repeated up to 10 times.

FIGURE 5. *A training program for home use.*

39

and the overcommitted man or woman should learn to reduce responsibility and cultivate contentment.

- Reduce dietary cholesterol and lipids. For years we've known that cholesterol contributes to atherosclerosis, and individuals with a cholesterol level greater than 250 mg per 100 ml have twice the risk of developing arteriosclerotic heart disease than individuals whose cholesterol is less than 220 mg per ml. For this reason, the American Heart Association recommends a daily cholesterol intake of about 300 mg, no easy task considering that one egg contains 275 mg of cholesterol and 4 oz. of meat about 120 mg of cholesterol. Plasma lipids have stolen the spotlight from cholesterol in recent years, and doctors have defined a number of specific abnormalities of blood lipids (fats). Specific diagnosis is possible only by blood tests including cholesterol (normal values about 150 to about 260 mg per ml). Even if no abnormality of cholesterol or lipids is present, restricting their intake can pay dividends in years to come. A low fat and cholesterol diet is found on Page 17.

A good source of further information about the prevention of atherosclerosis is:

The American Heart Association Inc.
7320 Greenville Avenue
Dallas, Texas 75231

BACKACHE

Synonyms: lower back strain, lumbago

Backache began when man first assumed the upright posture, placing an undue strain on the muscles supporting the lower spine. Bending forward from the waist, working in a stooped posture, or carrying heavy objects taxes the muscles and ligaments, sometimes beyond endurance, and low backache results. Sometimes back pain follows an acute injury or sudden strain, but more often it is the result of poor habits of lifting, standing, and sitting.

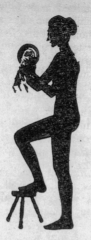

FIGURE 6. *One foot raised relaxes the lower back muscles.*

Preventing Lower Back Pain

Because of the origin of most backaches is postural, back strain can often be prevented by careful attention to habits in day-by-day activities. Here's a list of ten tips to help prevent muscular strain of the lower back;

- When reaching down, never bend from the waist; sit, squat, or kneel instead.
- When lifting, face the object, check your balance, think about your back, and bend both knees; use your strong thigh and shoulder muscles, keeping the back straight.
- Never move furniture, push a stalled car, or try to lift very heavy objects alone.
- Avoid prolonged standing whenever possible, but if you must stand at work, rest the back by elevating one foot on a hassock or footstool (see Figure 6).
- Women, avoid high heels in favor of firm walking shoes.
- Stay out of deep chairs and soft couches; your back prefers firm support.

41

- Sleep on your side, with one or both knees bent. If you feel you're only comfortable flat on your back, place a pillow under your knees. Sleeping on your stomach bows the back and should be avoided altogether.
- When driving, stop hourly and walk around the car to relax tension and loosen muscles.
- Stay slim; a protruding paunch is often balanced by painful swayback posture.
- Exercise daily to retain youthful muscle tone.

When Backache Strikes

Despite your best efforts, lower back pain may develop, with agonizing sapsm of the lower back muscles and difficulty in sleeping. For simple lower back strain, self-help therapy parallels what the doctor would advise: rest, heat, and medication.

Rest means getting off your feet. When severe lower back strain afflicts you, bed rest is advised. The most physiologic, and therefore the most comfortable position, is lying or sitting propped in bed with the knees bent, the same position you assume when in a reclining chair. Trips to the bathroom are allowed, but meals should be served in bed during the acute phase. With continued improvement, the patient is allowed to sit in a chair with the feet on a hassock. A tight lower back strain will keep most individuals home from work for three to seven days—sometimes longer (these patients should be checked by the doctor).

Heat brings blood into tight muscles and speeds healing. Moist heat is best: soak a towel in hot water, wring thoroughly, then apply the hot damp towel to the back. As it cools and dries, add more hot water. Be careful. Don't burn the skin. A hot water bottle or a heating pad are acceptable when there is no one at home to apply the hot packs. Heat should be applied for one hour, four times daily, and never, never sleep with a heating pad in place.

Medication relieves the pain of lower back strain. For most backaches, aspirin or acetaminophen (Tylenol) does the trick. Two tablets every six hours takes the edge off the pain and allows restful sleep. If that's not strong enough, the doctor may prescribe a combination muscle-relaxant and analgesic such as Parafon Forte containing the muscle relaxant chlorzoxazone (Paraflex) and acetaminophen (Tylenol). The pain-killer is continued until discomfort disappears.

Exercise helps loosen tight back muscles and strengthen supporting tissues of the spine. Figure 7 shows four exercises for low back pain (courtesy of McNeil Laboratories, Inc., Fort Washington, Pennsylvania).

Don't overdo exercising, especially in the beginning. Start by trying the movements slowly and carefully. If pain occurs and lasts more than 15 or 20 minutes, stop and do no further exercises until you see your doctor.

Do the exercises on a hard surface covered with a thin mat or heavy blanket. Put a pillow under your neck if it makes you more comfortable. Always start your exercises slowly—and in the order shown—to allow muscles to loosen up gradually. Heat treatments just before you begin can help relax tight muscles. Follow the instructions carefully; it will be well worth the effort.

Call the doctor promptly if the pain gets worse despite rest and heat, if the pain radiates down one leg (suggesting sciatica, a more troublesome disorder than simple low back strain), if there is numbness or weakness of an extremity, or if the pain persists for more than a week, (suggesting the possibility of a disorder other than simple low back strain).

BAD TRIP

Synonyms: acute hallucinosis, "bummer"

Most bad trips are due to LSD (D-lysergic acid diethylamide), although other mind-expanding drugs are sometimes indicated, including diethyltriptamine (DET), dimethyltriptamine (DMT), dimethyoxymethylamphetamine (DOM or STP), methylene dioxyamphetamine (MDA or the "love" drug), peyote, mescaline, certain mushrooms (psilocybin), or morning glory seeds (Rivera corimbosa).

The bad trip is terrifying, with distortion of reality, time, and thoughts. The victim's perception of sight and sound is intensified yet disrupted, and panic can result. The bad trip lasts for several hours or more, subsiding as the hallucinogen is metabolized. But occasionally the acute episode unmasks an emotional disorder previously held in check and persistent

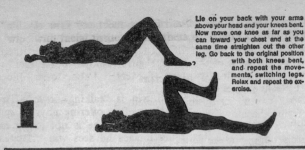

Lie on your back with your arms above your head and your knees bent. Now move one knee as far as you can toward your chest and at the same time straighten out the other leg. Go back to the original position with both knees bent, and repeat the movements, switching legs. Relax and repeat the exercise.

1

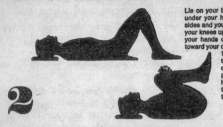

Lie on your back with a small pillow under your head, your arms at your sides and your knees bent. Now bring your knees up to your chest, and with your hands clasped pull your knees toward your chest. Hold for a count of 10, keeping your knees together and your shoulders flat on the mat. Repeat the pulling and holding movement three times. Relax and repeat the exercise.

2

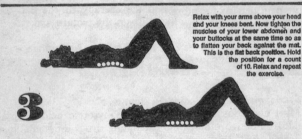

Relax with your arms above your head and your knees bent. Now tighten the muscles of your lower abdomen and your buttocks at the same time so as to flatten your back against the mat. This is the flat back position. Hold the position for a count of 10. Relax and repeat the exercise.

3

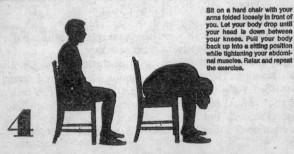

Sit on a hard chair with your arms folded loosely in front of you. Let your body drop until your head is down between your knees. Pull your body back up into a sitting position while tightening your abdominal muscles. Relax and repeat the exercise.

4

FIGURE 7. *Four exercises to strengthen the lower back.*

mental symptoms are seen. Occasionally reported are flash-backs or perceptual distortion occurring weeks or months after the bad trip.

Treating the Bad-Trip Victim

The treatment of the bad trip is "talking down." This means patiently sitting with the victim, offering physical and emotional support, reassuring him that he is not losing his mind and that the terrifying images he sees will disappear once the drug has left his system. He needs help coping with perceptual distortion—with identification of voices and localization of familiar objects in the room. Guilt is relieved by reassurance that his friends and family love him and will care for him during his present crisis.

A few cautions are in order: Don't make quick motions; they can be frightening. Beware of touching or holding the victim; it can be misconstrued as an attack. Be alert for the sudden attempt to escape via the door or window. Always try to remember that the bad-trip victim has temporarily lost his ability to perceive stimuli normally and to reason logically.

Medicine has little place in the therapy of the bad trip. Drug administration merely confuses the picture and may be harmful.

It is often helpful to call the physician for guidance, but the recognized therapy of the bad trip is sympathy rather than injections and patience instead of drugs.

BALDNESS

Synonym: alopecia

Baldness describes a loss of scalp hair, and may involve other areas of the body such as eyebrows and beard, or even a total absence of body hair. There may be a monk's ring of fringe around the scalp, a single bare island may be surrounded by a sea of wavy tresses, or the scalp may have a motheaten appearance. The pattern defines the type of baldness, and has implications concerning treatment.

Male-Pattern Baldness

My daughter just completed a school project in genetics, tracing early male-pattern baldness (a dominant trait) through six generations of our family and concluded that her father can blame his ancestors for his lack of hair.

Male-pattern baldness is characterized by hair loss, sometimes beginning in the teens and twenties, progressing to a dramatic top-of-the-head bald spot ringed by a crown of hair waiting its turn to depart. The forefathers of the affected individual usually suffered the same male-pattern baldness, and despite flawless grooming, scientific shampooing, and the nostrums sold by those who claim they can halt departing hair, the individual with a genetic predisposition to male-pattern baldness will eventually lose his hair.

Yet, self-help treatment may help delay the inevitable. Male hair loss may be associated with seborrhea of the scalp (see Dandruff) and treatment of this disorder may slow hair loss. A thyroid or vitamin deficiency may play a role, and correction of this defect can help preserve remaining hair. Hair abuse, with exposure to sun, wind, and extremes of temperature, as well as carelessly harsh combing and brushing can, hasten hair loss. Handle hair with care; as a wise man once said, "A hair in the head is worth two in the brush."

There's little else to be done for departing hair. And except for cosmetic surgery, the doctor has no more help to offer for male-pattern baldness. Self-help for this condition is best directed toward a change in mental attitude, accepting the rising forehead with equanimity and the shining pate with pride.

Alopecia Areata

A patchy hair loss characterizes alopecia areata, and bald spots may involve the scalp, eyebrows, eyelashes, or beard. The course is as unpredictable as the distribution, and spotty baldness may persist for months, years, or forever. The cause of alopecia areata is usually obscure, although emotional upheaval seems to play a role in many cases.

Patchy hair loss should be examined by the physician because, as we'll see, a treatable disease may be present. If the doctor confirms the diagnosis of alopecia areata, he may recommend injections of cortisone into the scalp, perhaps supplemented by the application of a cortisone lotion. These attempts sometimes fail, and sometimes succeed. The alternative is to await hopefully and expectantly the regrowth of hair.

Alopecia of Pregnancy

Here's a type of hair loss that doesn't need the doctor's care. Ask your local beautician; she'll confirm that two or three months after delivery, or perhaps following anesthesia, women often lose hair by the handful. Self-help treatment includes gentle hair care, brushing and combing judiciously to minimize tugging at hair roots. Permanents and color treatments should be deferred until hair has regrown, and the best shampoo choice is an extra-mild product such as Allercreme Soap Shampoo.

Finally, the most important self-help treatment of all is reassurance. Almost without fail, hair lost following pregnancy will regrow within a few months, regaining its previous texture and fullness.

Traction Alopecia

Tight hair styles that tug at the temples cause traction hair loss, often seen in the teenager with a ponytail hairdo.

The only treatment necessary is finding a new hair style, one that doesn't pull at the hair roots.

Hot Comb Alopecia

Women who straighten kinky hair with hot combs suffer a distinctive type of hair loss. The only therapy that works is stopping hot comb use. Fortunately, with Afro hair styles in vogue, hot comb alopecia is becoming much less common.

Hair Loss Due to Disease

Alopecia may be a first hint of illness, and that's why unusual or persistent hair loss should be examined by a physician. A thyroid deficiency causes dry, thinning hair, sometimes associated with a loss of eyebrow hair. Ringworm causes one or more bald patches, and a moth-eaten scalp characterizes advanced syphilis. Then there are medications that can cause baldness, including colchicine, heparin, coumarin; plus certain anticancer drugs and x-ray therapy.

BED-WETTING

Synonym: enuresis

Enuresis is why Mary won't go to slumber parties and David shuns summer camp. Although neither painful nor fatal, bed-wetting is nevertheless a source of monumental anguish to the afflicted youngster.

Let's start at the beginning: All infants have enuresis, and by the age of one year the youngster becomes aware of the sensation of a full bladder. By his second birthday the child usually learns to control urination during daytime hours, and by age three is usually dry day and night, although sporadic bed-wetting may occur until ages four or even five.

Nighttime urinary control comes when the bladder can hold comfortably about 10 ounces or urine—the child's urinary production between night and morning. Until this capacity is achieved, enuresis will occur.

Coping with Bed-Wetting

Since bed-wetting is more or less normal in preschool youngsters, it's vital that guilt feelings not be imparted. Praise success, but don't condemn the child for his occasional accident. Be patient; almost all cases of enuresis are self-limited (unless disease is present), and bed-wetting will subside eventually—whether because of or in spite of treatment.

Restricting fluids from supper until bedtime and awakening Mary or Johnny when Mommy and Daddy retire is a time-honored ritual in enuresis. Usually it is of little help.

A wind-up alarm clock sometimes helps older children achieve nighttime urinary control. The child is awakened, the bladder is emptied, and the alarm is reset ahead another two hours. In time, the interval is lengthened progressively until the child is asleep and dry all night.

A useful self-help method aims to increase bladder capacity. Here's how: Encourage the child to hold urine during the day for as long as comfortably possible. Then measure the urinary output. It may take months, but when the bladder volume reaches 10 to 12 ounces, nighttime urinary control often develops.

Some parents use a wet-bed alarm, available through most pharmacies. The first drop of urine connects an electrical circuit, activating an alarm device. The child is awakened abruptly, and hopefully is conditioned to associate the need to void with a nocturnal trip to the toilet.

Bed-Wetting and the Physician

If enurèsis persists past the sixth birthday, the physician should be consulted for two reasons. First, up to 10 percent of youngsters with persistent bed-wetting have disorders of the urinary system. If present, a urologic abnormality can cause permanent bladder or kidney damage unless it is diagnosed and treated during childhood. Second, the doctor has available medications that may break the bed-wedding cycle.

Once he has excluded infection or other urinary abnormalities, the doctor may prescribe imipramine (Tofranil), one tablet taken at bedtime to help prevent bed-wetting. Or the prescription may be for an atropine compound (to help inhibit urination during the night), or for ephedrine (to lighten the level of sleep).

In the final analysis, hard-core bed-wetters without evidence of physical disease may respond only to psychological counseling, increased maturity, and the passage of time.

BELCHING

Synonyms: eructation, burping

A bubble of gas in the stomach may rise up the esophagus and escape with an audible "burp" at the most inopportune times. Some persons belch only when anxious; others associate eructation with certain foods, with gulped meals, carbonated beverages, and/or gum chewing. In all cases, belching is caused by gas trapped in the stomach, which escapes to bring relief (and sometimes embarrassment).

Overcoming Belching

Relaxed mealtimes, with thorough chewing of food, minimize air swallowing and hence belching. Some foods—beans, cucumbers, radishes, and cabbage—may provoke belching, and these should be avoided, as should carbonated drinks.

If belching is simply a symptom of anxiety, it's time to lower life's stresses, perhaps reducing responsibility, and curbing conflicts. An occasional individual swallows air while chewing gum, nibbling candy, or inhaling (and swallowing) tobacco smoke. Elimination of these habits helps overcome eructation.

Pay attention to your swallowing mechanism. If you are anxiously gulping air, or acquiring a stomach bubble while eating or smoking, self-help care can eliminate eructation.

Medication sometimes helps. An old-time remedy is rhubarb and soda, taken as a dose of two teaspoonfuls after each meal. A more modern remedy is simethicone (Mylicon)—one 80-mg tablet chewed after each meal to reduce troublesome gas and belching.

BELL'S PALSY

Synonym: facial-nerve palsy

At first blush, Bell's palsy looks like a stroke, but its implications are much less ominous. The onset is usually sudden, and the victim awakes one morning to notice one side of the face drooping into a grotesque caricature. There may be difficulty closing the eye and there may be drooling from the corner of the mouth.

The cause of Bell's palsy is often obscure, although sometimes there is disease of the middle ear, such as an ear infection, causing pressure on the nerve to the facial muscles as it passes nearby. Bell's palsy is thus a paralysis of the muscles of one side of the face, occurring in the absence of weakness of the extremities or other sign of stroke.

Treatment

Suspected Bell's palsy should be examined by the doctor, allowing the option of initiating cortisone treatment or formal physical therapy. Nevertheless, self-help treatment can do much:

- Massage, using a light fingertip motion, stimulates nerve fibers and increases blood flow. Do it gently for 10 to 15 minutes four times daily.
- Passive exercise also uses a light fingertip motion, moving the weakened muscles to preserve mobility.
- Active exercises begin when strength starts to return. Forcibly wrinkling the forehead, closing the eye, and baring the teeth help move the facial muscles through their full range of motion; repeat 10 times each, four times daily.
- An eye patch may be applied at bedtime (and perhaps also during waking hours) to prevent damage to the cornea when muscular weakness prevents closing the eye.

Most, but not all, cases of Bell's palsy recover eventually. Some take six weeks, and some six months to achieve facial symmetry. Unfortunately, a few individuals (particularly the elderly) never recover the full use of facial muscles following an attack of Bell's palsy.

BLINDNESS

Impaired vision afflicts more than three million Americans, and many have been declared legally blind—unable to read 20/200 (the big E on the eye chart) even with corrective lenses.

Blindness comes from many causes, including hereditary defects, childhood injuries (or for that matter trauma at any age), infection of the cornea, glaucoma, or even the administration of excessive doses of oxygen to newborn infants.

The self-help therapy of blindness is prevention, avoiding possible causes and staying alert for dangers that may threaten vision.

Preserving Visual Acuity

Here are seven tips to help preserve vision:

- Never allow children to play with sharp-pointed toys,

air rifles, and arrows—unless under strict adult supervision.

- Foreign bodies in the eye should be removed only by a physician, especially if imbedded in the cornea (the clear area over the pupil and iris).
- When using machinery that may emit dust or sparks, use safety glasses to protect the eyes.
- Contact lenses may cause infection. Avoid contamination by careful handwashing before insertion, thorough cleansing of the lens in an antiseptic solution before and after use, and limited use of contact lenses, since prolonged retention of the lens may lead to irritation.
- Blindness due to congenital rubella is prevented by administration of live rubella virus vaccine to all susceptible females, as discussed on page 267.
- See the doctor about all red or painful eyes. The disorder may be simple pinkeye, but more serious conditions such as iritis and glaucoma must not be overlooked.
- Have your vision (and that of your children) tested each year, particularly if there is frequent blinking, difficulty in performing close work, blurred or double vision, headaches, or other symptoms that may be linked to visual problems.

Help for the Visually Handicapped

The treatment and prevention of blindness are the aims of several organizations engaged in research, education, and service at the local level. Further information can be obtained by writing to:

National Society for the Prevention of Blindness, Inc.
79 Madison Avenue
New York, New York 10016

Fight for Sight, Inc.
National Council to Combat Blindness, Inc.
41 West 57th Street
New York, New York 10019

National Aid to Visually Handicapped
3201 Balboa Street
San Francisco, California 94121

American Foundation for the Blind, Inc.
15 West 16th Street
New York, New York 10011

Research to Prevent Blindness, Inc.
598 Madison Avenue
New York, New York 10022

BODY ODOR

Heeding the message of television advertisements, Americans of all ages worry about body odor. In fact, fresh sweat—containing water and salt—is odorless, although an odor may follow if the evaporation of perspiration is impeded by warm body folds or occlusive clothing, and bacterial growth begins.

Deodorants and antiperspirants are useful in the underarms. Deodorants contain antiseptics that inhibit bacterial growth—the true culprit in body odor—while antiperspirants contain aluminum salts to decrease sweat formation.

The following procedures may help to allay apprehension about body odor:

- Bathe or shower thoroughly each morning, using an unscented soap such as Ivory. Rinse thoroughly to remove all the soap residue, then dry briskly.
- Pay special attention to thorough drying of the underarms, groin, and rectal areas, where moist skin folds favor bacterial growth.
- Powder lightly with nonmedicated talcum powder, being sure to include skin fold areas.
- Apply an antiperspirant to the underarms.
- Be sure all body areas and the antiperspirant have dried before dressing.
- Whenever possible, wear loosely fitting, well-ventilated clothes to facilitate the evaporation of normal body perspiration.

BOTULISM

Three percent of reported food poisonings in the United States are due to clostridium botulinus, which carries a terrifying mortality of about 50 percent in untreated patients. Bacteria growing in improperly preserved foods produce a toxin that impairs nerve function. Early symptoms are indistinguishable from other types of food poisoning: diarrhea, nausea, vomiting, and a burning abdominal pain. Then follow dizziness, dry mouth, blurred vision, impaired swallowing, slurred speech, and muscular weakness. Symptoms usually begin within two days of eating the contaminated food and death may occur within one week.

Self-help measures include the proper preservation and serving of foods, plus the recognition of possible botulism.

Don't even sample potentially contaminated foods, since a tiny taste of botulinus toxin can cause serious consequences. Discard without opening food cans whose ends are ballooned by possible fermentation within. Canned or preserved foods that smell spoiled should also be discarded. Foods canned domestically should be boiled four to six hours before sealing.

Botulinus toxin is destroyed by heat, and home-preserved foods should be boiled at least five minutes before serving.

If symptoms of food poisoning (or what may seem to be a viral gastroenteritis) progress to involve speech, vision, and motor nerves, call the doctor immediately. Botulinus antitoxin may be lifesaving and, although not routinely available in most hospitals, it may be obtained from the National Communicable Disease Center, Atlanta, Georgia (telephone: (404) 633-3311 or (404) 663-2176).

BRONCHITIS

Synonyms: bronchial infection, chest congestion

Bronchitis means inflammation of the bronchial tubes and it is an affliction shared by millions of Americans. The universal symptom is a cough—sometimes dry and hacking, sometimes productive of gray or yellow sputum. With the cough there may be a coarse clearing of the throat, occasional wheezing and shortness of breath, and perhaps weight loss due to advanced disease. These symptoms of bronchitis can usually be traced to some combination of allergy, irritation, and infection.

Allergy contributes to many cases of chronic bronchitis as susceptible individuals develop bronchial irritation upon inhaling plant pollen, house dust, animal dander, or airborne molds. Sometimes symptoms are seasonal—as grass-allergic individual cough most during the spring of the year or the individual allergic to animal dander may improve during summer when Rover stays outdoors.

Irritation due to exhaust fumes and industrial pollutants plays a major role in bronchitis, both in America and in the industrial centers of other countries. This fact notwithstanding, the chief irritant indicated in bronchitis is tobacco smoke. Even the smoke from a cigarette enjoyed by another in the room can cause bronchial irritation in a susceptible individual.

Infection seeks out chronically irritated membranes, and it is not long before bronchi inflamed by allergy and/or irritation develop colonies of bacteria. Mucus and phlegm are produced as the battle against infection rages, causing a cough that produecs sputum.

The Battle against Bronchitis

Bronchitis is attacked on three fronts. Allergy-provoking substances are avoided whenever possible. Eliminate dust-catching rugs, Venetian blinds, and nicknacks from the house. If the family dog or cat is proven to be causing allergic bronchitis, the animal must be banished from the household. When feasible, an electrostatic air filter, and perhaps an air conditioner, is installed to remove circulating allergens from household air.

Stopping smoking eliminates the prime source of bronchial irritation, and others in the household should be discouraged from smoking in the presence of a chronic bronchitis sufferer. Individuals with chronic cough and chest congestion who reside in a smog area should consider moving to a less polluted site.

Infection calls for antibiotics, and this means a trip to the doctor's office for therapy. Often prescribed is tetracycline, one 250-mg tablet taken four times daily. In chronic cases, the antibiotic may be taken three or four days weekly with rest periods in between.

Expectorants help dissolve sticky phlegm deep in the bronchi. An over-the-counter favorite is glyceryl guaiacolate (Robitussin), one teaspoon taken four times daily to liquefy thick mucus. If chronic cough is a problem, the doctor may prescribe a cough syrup containing codeine to help clear the bronchial tubes while suppressing an exhausting and unproductive cough.

Postural drainage helps drain phlegm from hidden recesses of the lungs. Here's how it's done. Take two teaspoonfuls of glyceryl guaiacolate, followed by a full glass of water to help start mucus moving. Then lie over the side of the bed, face down—legs and hips on the bed, elbows and forearms on the floor (see Figure 8). With the head dependent, cough several times to start the mucus flowing downhill; turn to the right, then to the left, to clear mucus from trapped pockets.

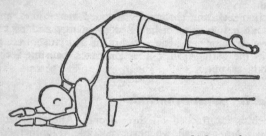

FIGURE 8. *Postural drainage of bronchial secretions: waist at edge of bed, weight on elbows and forearms on floor.*

All but the most stubborn cases of bronchitis can be alleviated by these measures, an important consideration since untreated chronic bronchitis can lead to pulmonary emphysema (see Emphysema).

BRUISE

Synonyms: contusion, blunt injury
A bruise occurs when you stub a toe, bump a hip on furni-

ture, or fall and land on an elbow. There's local pain and perhaps a black-and-blue mark, but the skin is intact.

If there is no laceration and no bone broken, self-help therapy should suffice. Here's the basic theory of treating bruises of all areas: Apply ice for the first 24 hours, to reduce swelling. After 24 hours, switch the applications to heat. Moist compresses are best for both cold and hot applications, and are applied for 30 to 60 minutes four times daily. Rest for the injured area is helpful, especially if an extremity is involved; a sling or Ace elastic bandage is often used.

Larger black-and-blue areas, called ecchymoses, may take several weeks to clear, and occasionally blood cells form a persistent (but otherwise harmless) fibrous lump of scar tissue beneath the skin.

BUNION

A bunion is a partial dislocation at the base of the great toe. It usually follows years of wearing cramped footwear, perhaps aggravated by long hours on the feet, and made worse if high heels force the weight down onto the toes and ball of the foot. In time the deformed joint becomes swollen and painful and walking becomes a chore.

How to Help the Bunion

Because most bunions can be traced to improper footwear, ill-fitting shoes should be discarded. Perhaps the wearer needs a half or full size wider shoe, perhaps a size longer. Discard high heels in favor of low-heeled, sturdy footwear, and minimize walking until pain disappears.

Acute discomfort often responds to hot compresses applied for 30 minutes four times daily. When sleeping, strapping may help reduce the dislocation or a bunion brace may be worn to help restore proper alignment.

In the end, many bunions come to surgery to abolish the pain and restore a normal contour to the joint.

BURNS

A burn is a thermal injury to skin and perhaps deeper structures. The source may be hot coffee, charcoal embers, the red-hot exhaust pipe on a motorcycle, or any of a hundred other sources of thermal energy.

Doctors classify burns according to degree: A first-degree burn causes redness of the skin and severe pain, but no blisters are present. Blistering characterizes the second-degree burn, which is also quite painful and may progress to infection. A third-degree burn chars all layers of the skin; it may be painless because of destroyed nerve endings, and usually requires skin grafts for closure.

Treament

When a burn occurs, prompt home treatment helps reduce tissue damage. The burned area should be plunged instantly into cold water—neutralizing the effect of heat and removing any residual hot coffee, smoldering embers, etc. Maintain the application of cold water for 30 minutes, then examine the burn.

If the area is small—only a few inches in diameter—and shows no evidence of blistering, then you're dealing with a first-degree burn. No particular therapy is needed after the initial immersion in cold water. Overcome the urge to smear it with butter or lard; leave the area open to the air, and continue to observe for blisters that may form a few hours later.

Superficial burns often respond nicely to the application of the watery gel of the Aloe Vera plant. The tropical Aloe Vera plant grows in your garden if you live in Florida or on your kitchen window sill if you live "up north." When a small burn occurs, cut off a shoot an inch or two long and squeeze the plant's jelly directly onto the burn. There's fast relief of pain, and prompt healing. In addition, Vitamin C helps heal burns. Take 3,000 to 4,000 mg daily for one week to aid healing.

Blistered burns are second-degree, and these should usually be covered to avoid infection. If more than a few square inches of skin surface are involved, or if the burn has occurred on a difficult-to-bandage or sensitive area such as the web between the fingers or the skin of the face, then it's best to visit a physician. He'll apply a snug dressing over a layer of white petrolatum (Vaseline) or mafenide (Sulfamylon) cream. Several changes of dressing, at three or four-day intervals, are usually needed, and sometimes the doctor trims away dead skin enclosing blisters.

A second-degree burn involving a small area of easy-to-bandage skin, such as on the forearm, can be treated at home. After immersion in cold water, cleanse the area very gently with soap and water, then rinse and dry. Apply a thin layer of nonprescription Bacitracin Ointment to retard infection and to prevent your dressing from sticking. Next comes a nonstick Telfa Pad, covered by 4 × 4-inch bandages held securely in place with nonallergenic adhesive tape such as Dermicel Tape. Replace the self-help dressing every day and call the doctor promptly if increasing pain, drainage of pus, or a foul odor signals infection.

After immersion in cold water, third-degree burns require professional medical treatment. Keep covered with cold compresses while on your way to the doctor or hospital. Recommended may be soaks with a silver nitrate solution, perhaps followed by skin grafting.

The doctor will recommend a tetanus booster for victims of third-degree and second-degree burns if one has not been administered within the last few years.

Preventing Burns

- Keep a home fire extinguisher close at hand; make sure it will work when needed; have the pressure checked annually.
- Prevent electrical burns of toddlers by shielding unused electrical outlets.
- When cooking hot liquids on the stovetop, keep the handles turned toward the wall rather than protruding where they can be struck while you're walking by.
- Don't let gasoline- or turpentine-soaked rags accumulate in the basement workshop.
- Repair frayed electrical cords promptly.
- Be careful with hot coffee or tea when children are around.
- Keep matches out of the reach of youngsters.

CANCER

Synonyms: carcinoma, neoplasm, malignant tumor

Cancer describes a malignant growth that can arise in almost any organ of the body and that, if unchecked, can grow to destroy vital tissue and cause death. Trailing only cardiovascular disease, cancer is the number-two cause of death in America today.

What is Cancer?

Cancer is a growth of cells gone wild. Beginning in a previously normal organ such as the lung or brain, or even in bone, cancer produces new mutant cells that multiply rapidly and soon overrun the normal tissues. Sometimes cancer causes pressure on nearby vital structures, while other tumor cells may migrate to distant parts of the body. Virtually any organ in the body can develop cancer, with symptoms, physical findings, and microscopic features peculiar to that tumor. By definition, malignant tumors cause death when untreated, and benign tumors may impair nearby organs, but without fatal termination.

From observations made over centuries, we know five factors that favor the development of cancer:

- Heredity may have an influence. Racial traits and family susceptibility account for the occurrence of the same cancer in identical twins. Certain strains of mice predictably develop specific cancers in each generation. Blacks rarely suffer malignant melanoma of the skin, Caucasians develop cancer of the prostate nine times as often as Japanese, and Chinese have a high incidence of cancer of the nasopharynx—all related to heredity, or perhaps to some factor as yet unknown.

- Carcinogens, substances that incite cancer, are factors that we can control. Potential carcinogens include hydrocarbon derivatives, coal dust, paraffin oil, aniline dyes, tobacco smoke, cyclamates, asbestos, x-rays, and radioactive material. The carcinogenic properties of carbon soot were recognized in 1775 when Dr. Percival Potts noted the frequent occurence of scrotal cancer in young boys working as chimney sweeps. Fishermen who mend their nets with tarred twine, holding it in the mouth, have a sky-high incidence of lip cancer. Icelanders suffer a high frequency of stomach cancer, probably related to a diet high in smoked meats and fish. Bladder cancer occurs in aniline dye workers more often than in the general population, and x-ray specialists suffer leukemia ten times more frequently than other individuals.

- Hormones play a role in certain cancers, notably of breast and prostate, both of which grow luxuriantly under hormonal stimulation. And in 1976 medical studies linked estrogen hormones to endometrial cancer of the uterus.
- Viruses may be the missing link in cancer. In some tumors of chickens the evidence appears conclusive. Microorganisms may be the answer to why early circumcision protects adult males from cancer of the penis and their wives from cervical cancer. The Epstein-Barr virus of infectious mononucleosis has been linked to malignant lymphoma.
- Preexisting disease may lead to cancer growth. Skin cancers are common in old burn scars; the alcoholic is particularly at risk for cancer of the esophagus and larynx; and more than half of all liver tumors (hepatomas) strike adults with cirrhosis of the liver.

Where Cancer Strikes

Most cancers occur in individuals in their fifties and sixties. The reason is simple: this is the largest age group at risk. During later decades, deaths from diseases of old age lower the number of cancer cases reported, as individuals who might have developed cancer succumb to heart attacks, strokes, and so on. For the individual, however, the risk of developing most cancers increases with age.

Death due to cancers of various types is linked not so much to the incidence of the tumor as to its malignancy. Malignant tumors metastasize—spread from the original site to distant organs, often giving rise to widely scattered secondary growths. Therein lies the lethal threat of cancer.

The following are the most common causes of cancer deaths in males:

1. Lung cancer, conclusively linked to excessive cigarette smoking, leads the list.
2. Colon and rectum cancers, many detectable by physical and x-ray examinations, and curable if found early.
3. Prostate cancer, common in older males.
4. Stomach cancer, often causing the same symptoms as ulcer.
5. Pancreas cancer, deep in the abdomen and hard to detect.

Women have their own special cancer problems. Here are the five leading causes of female cancer deaths:

1. Breast cancer, most common between ages 45 and 65, uncommon after 65; yet 17 percent of cases occur in women under 40 years of age.
2. Colon and rectum cancers, the most frequent internal "non-feminine" tumors of women, often cause rectal bleeding and changes in bowel habit.
3. Cancer of the uterus and cervix, also striking a younger age group than many other tumors. The tip-off is often a questionable Papanicolaou smear upon routine pelvic examination.
4. Cancer of the ovary, nestled deep in the pelvis, often eludes detection until well advanced.
5. Lung cancer, increasing in incidence each year.

Cancer is the second leading cause of death (following accidents) in children, and the tumors suffered by youngsters tend to be rapid-growing and malignant. The five leading types of fatal cancers of children are:

1. Leukemia, with combination chemotherapy now showing promise of some cures.
2. Brain, one of the most feared of all tumors.
3. Lymphosarcoma, the object of some hopeful scientific experiments.
4. Kidney, often detected too late to cure.

5. Bone, a tumor of youngsters that achieved notoriety when it struck Senator Edward Kennedy's son.

Diagnosis of Cancer

Until the riddle of cancer is solved and the doctor can offer a shot to treat or even to prevent the disease, our best defense is early detection and therapy. Here's where self-help can really pay off, with prompt recognition of possible early evidence of tumors.

The American Cancer Society and doctors have helped publicize the warning signs of cancer:

- A sore that does not heal, suggesting a neoplasm (a new, abnormal tissue growth) of skin or mucus membranes.
- A lump or thickening in the breast or other area, perhaps the first sign of tumor growth.
- A change in a mole or a wart, which may signal malignant deterioration of a skin lesion.
- Unusual discharge or bleeding, suspicious signs that scream for investigation of the involved organ.
- Persistent indigestion or difficulty in swallowing, which may be the clue to cancer of the throat, esophagus, or stomach.
- Persistent cough or hoarseness, possible signs of cancer of the respiratory organs.
- A change in bowel habits, which may mean cancer of the rectum or colon.
- Unexplained weight loss or prolonged fever—ominous signs that may occur with almost any type of tumor.

If cancer is suspected, call the doctor promptly. Two-thirds of all cancers can be cured if treated early. The physician will pin down the proper diagnosis, and if a tumor is present it will be attacked with surgery, radiation, or chemical therapy. Each day hundreds of individuals ignore cancer's warning signs and allow malignancies to persist past the time of total cure. Help yourself and your doctor fight cancer by promptly evaluating all suspicious physical symptoms.

If you are interested in learning more about cancer—whether your question concerns detection, home care, medical treatment available, or what's new in research—write to:

American Cancer Society, Inc.
219 East 42nd Street
New York, New York 10017
(One informative publication to request is "The Hopeful
Side of Cancer.")

Damon Runyon Memorial Fund for Cancer Research,
Inc.
33 West 56th Street
New York, New York 10019

CANDIDIASIS

Synonyms: moniliasis, yeast infection

Candida albicans is a ubiquitous infection occurring in the mouths of infants (where it is called thrush), in the vaginas of adult women (especially common in women taking birth control pills), and in skin folds of the body (including the underarms, groin, and the recesses under heavy breasts).

As you might guess, Candida organisms like warm, moist areas. They're often present on the skin, but begin to multiply and cause infection when resistance is lowered during a cold or flu, when the host is diabetic, or when antibiotic use upsets the ecological balance of skin organisms.

Once a toehold is gained, Candida germs spread, causing a beefy purple-red and often slightly shiny skin rash, surrounded by small satellite colonies and intensely itchy. If present in the infant's mouth, white material not unlike milk curds is seen. Vaginal infections have severe itching, with pain upon attempted sexual relations, plus a thick white discharge and involvement of nearby skin.

Treatment

The therapy of yeast infections is governed by the affected area. For generations, infants with oral thrush have been treated by swabbing the mouth with gentian violet four times daily; it's an unsightly treatment, but it still works and may be prescribed by the physician if therapy mentioned below fails. Beside local therapy, nursing-bottle nipples and pacifiers must be carefully sterilized and indolent pacifier sucking (which can stimulate germ growth) is prohibited.

When candidal infections strike skin folds, better ventilation is needed. Nylon underwear should be discarded in favor of cotton, and loose garments worn to promote air circulation. After washing, thoroughly dry infected areas, and a talcum dusting powder helps absorb moisture. Underarm shaving, which may allow infection to enter tiny nicks and cuts, is discouraged until the infection is cleared.

Vaginal yeast infections are often linked with tampon use, yet some women with copious candidal vaginal secretions have used tampons daily for weeks—trying to control their discharge while in fact making the infection worse by introducing a foreign body into the infected area. Instead of tampons, perineal pads (sanitary napkins) are advised. Also helpful may be douching with Massengill's Power—two rounded teaspoonfuls in a quart of warm water, mixed thoroughly—done two or three times weekly.

Nevertheless, these self-help measures will almost always fail unless specific anticandidal prescription therapy is used. Most often recommended is nystatin (Mycostatin)—available as an oral solution for thrush, a cream for skin infections, and insertable tablets to use for vaginal infections due to candidiasis.

CARDIAC ARREST

Synonym: heart stoppage

If cardiac arrest has occurred and you're reading now to find out what to do, it is already too late. When the heartbeat stops, instant action is needed, because more than four minutes without adequate blood-borne oxygen can cause permanent brain damage. Knowing in advance what to do when the heartbeat stops can someday save a life.

Diagnosis and Treatment

- Diagnose cardiac arrest by feeling the pulse and listening for the heartbeat. The patient may be gasping for breath or not moving at all, and the skin will look both pale and slightly blue (cyanosis, due to lack of oxygen in the blood). Once you're sure the heart has stopped, send a bystander for medical aid and begin resuscitation immediately.

- A sharp blow to the sternum (breastbone) with the clenched fist sometimes restores the normal heart rhythm. In practice it rarely works, but it's quick, reasonably safe, and deserves a try.
- Assisted ventilation means breathing for the victim. Air is needed in the lungs to boost the oxygen level in the bloodstream. Mouth-to-mouth ventilation is the accepted method. With the patient lying on his back, use one hand to depress the tongue with your thumb, while tilting the chin up to extend the neck. With the other hand, pinch his nostrils to prevent air leakage. Then take a deep breath, cover the patient's mouth with yours (also cover the nose if the victim is a child), and exhale forcefully, watching his chest rise from the corner of your eye. Continue breathing for the victim at about 12 breaths per minute until professional help arrives. (A fuller description of this procedure is found under Resuscitation.)
- Cardiac resuscitation stimulates blood circulation by manually compressing and releasing the heart. Lay the patient face up on a firm surface—the floor is fine. Kneel to the side and place the heel of one hand over the lower breastbone, the other hand on top of the first. Apply vigorous pressure, toward the spine, then release rapidly; the correct rate is about 60 beats per minute. If you're alone, coordinate the heart rate with breathing, by alternating five chest compressions for one mouth-to-mouth breath.
- Don't give up too soon. Continue resuscitation until the patient is fully awake or until you are relieved by a medical professional.

CARDIAC ARRHYTHMIA

The cardiac arrhythmias are disorders of the heart's rhythm. Included are arterial fibrillation (a total irregularity of the heartbeat), atrial flutter (a short-circuiting of the electrical impulses of the heart), skipped beats of the heart (often described as palpitation), paroxysmal atrial tachycardia (distinct episodes of very rapid heartbeat that begin and end abruptly, and more. All must be diagnosed by the physician following physical examination and electrocardiography, and may be treated by medicines such as digitalis, propranolol (Inderal), quinidine, or others.

To help to prevent cardiac irregularities and aid your doctor's treatment:

- Don't smoke.
- Stay slim, and avoid heavy meals.
- Sidestep emotional turmoil and minimize responsibility that may cause anxiety.
- Get plenty of relaxation, including rest periods during the day and a full eight hours of sleep each night.
- Take frequent vacations to "recharge your batteries."
- Don't take coffee, tea, or other stimulants.
- Don't take medications, even over-the-counter preparations, unless approved by the physician.
- Follow your doctor's instructions to the letter.

CATARACT

Synonym: cloudy lens of the eye

One of the ills of aging is the cataract—a cloudiness of the eye's lens that causes a gradual but progressive diminution in vision. A family tendency is common, and diabetics suffer more than their share of cataracts. If you sense diminished vision, see the doctor. He'll diagnose the cataract following an examination with the ophthalmoscope, an instrument for viewing the eye's interior. If a cloudy lens prevents light rays from reaching the retina, the doctor will be able to see through the opaque lens.

When "ripe," the cataract is treated surgically. The lens may be removed, although a new surgical development destroys the opaque lens with ultrasonic waves. Following surgery, corrective lenses (perhaps as contact lenses) will be prescribed.

Correct timing of surgery takes judgment, and I often advise patients that their cataracts are ready for definitive treatment when their failing vision hampers their activities, whether fishing, playing golf, reading, or watching the cars go by.

CEREBRAL PALSY

Synonyms: birth injury, Little's disease

Cerebral palsy follows brain injury at birth. Sometimes the disability can be traced to a rapid and traumatic delivery, the overenthusiastic use of forceps, or a difficult childbirth due to breach or other abnormal position of the infant. Sometimes the delivery seems normal as apple pie, yet the infant fails to breathe for a few minutes after birth, resulting a deficient oxygen supply to the brain.

No single defect characterizes cerebral palsy, and victims may show paralysis of the extremities, tightened muscles (spastic paraylsis), or mental defects. Weakness of the limbs is caused by damage to the brain and cannot be corrected. Nevertheless, exercises can strengthen intact nearby muscles and sometimes surgery is indicated to stabilize weakened joints.

Helping the Victim of Cerebral Palsy

The child with cerebral palsy may require special training, physical therapy, and braces, plus loads of patience and love.

Special appliances and braces can minimize the impact of weakened muscles, helping stabilize ankle and knee joints that otherwise could not bear weight. Walking may be aided by crutches, either conventional or of the Canadian type (with forearm braces).

Exercise has two goals: strengthening functioning muscle groups and preventing muscle contractures, with attendant joint tightness. Each joint and muscle group of an involved extremity should be exercised at least twice daily. Active exercise uses functioning muscles and builds strength. Following a period of active exercise, each joint in the extremity should be passively moved through its full range of motion several times. In addition, the patient should be encouraged to keep the foot flat (rather than pointing the toes) and the knees straight (raher than flexed) whenever possible; this helps avoid muscle tightening that can magnify the disability of cerebral palsy.

Special training can help youngsters and their parents compensate for disabilities, helping them cope with the activities of daily living, and perhaps offering vocational guidance. Some parents hesitate to enroll their child in the CP program, fearing that a stigma may be attached to the youngster. By doing so, they deny the child vital training that could aid him in the years to come.

Helpful information may be obtained from either of these two sources:

United Cerebral Palsy Associations, Inc.
66 East 34th Street
New York, New York 10016

National Society for Crippled Children and Adults, Inc.
2023 West Ogden Avenue
Chicago, Illinois 60610

CHICKEN POX

Synonym: varicella

The name chicken pox comes from the word chickpea, roughly descriptive of the typical skin lesion but of scant interest to the youngster suffering this disorder's intense itching. Following an incubation period of about two weeks, the victim develops a low-grade fever and fatigue, followed by successive crops of pox—teardrop-like blisters on a bright red base that, when scratched, break to form a crusted surface. The most common complication is infection developing in one or more of the skin pox.

Treatment

Let's start by saying that nothing need be done. Chicken pox is a self-limited disease and, in the absence of all treatment, will subside within about one week—with lesions crusted and healing and the child probably ready to return to school. Self-help treatment of chicken pox is directed toward relieving symptoms, plus preventing or treating the occasional infection.

Fever is treated with aspirin, although large doses are rarely necessary since high fevers are uncommon with chicken pox. Nevertheless, an occasional dose of aspirin (maximum: one grain of aspirin per year of age to top dose of 10 grains— taken every six to eight hours) may help relieve itching.

Cleanliness can help prevent many infections, and I recommend that my chicken pox patients take a thorough tub bath daily, including an all-over scrub with Ivory Soap and a thorough rinse with clean water. Occasionally you'll hear the old wives' tale that bathing makes chicken pox worse; don't believe it. Severe itching may respond to Alpha-Keri Water Dispersible Antipruritic Oil—one to two capfuls in a bathtub of water. Some mothers insist that the best relief comes with an Aveeno Colloidal Oatmeal Bath.

Local therapy of intensely itching chicken pox provides symptomatic relief, and gives the child a feeling that something is being done. Try small spot applications of Calamine Lotion with 0.5 percent menthol or perhaps plain Lubriderm Lotion. For intense itching, call the doctor and suggest a prescription antipruritic medication such as methdilazine (Tacaryl) chewable tablets or syrup.

Neosporin Ointment is used for infected pox. When bacteria cause pus, soreness, and increasing redness, scrub with Ivory soap, dry, then apply Neosporin Ointment four times daily. Most superficial skin infections resolve promptly, although occasional scarring is seen.

Return to school is delayed until all lesions show evidence of healing—usually about seven days after the appearance of the first pock.

CIRRHOSIS OF THE LIVER

Synonyms: portal cirrhosis, Laennec's cirrhosis, alcoholic cirrhosis

Cirrhosis is a chronic liver disease characterized by loss of appetite, weakness, and constant fatigue, leading inevitably to jaundice, abdominal swelling, weight loss, and eventual liver failure.

In most instances portal cirrhosis follows chronic alcoholism linked with malnutrition, as the alcoholic individual consumes several thousand fuel calories in whiskey, wine, or even beer each day. Burning alcohol as fuel, he has neither the appetite nor the funds for vitamin-rich food, and multiple dietary deficiencies develop.

What to Do about Cirrhosis

For the heavy drinker-poor eater, let there be no confusion about the advice offered here: The self-help plan for preventing and treating cirrhosis includes eating better and drinking not at all.

This means nutritious meals including fresh fruit, meat, vegetables, and dairy products plus a supplementary multivitamin (such as Optilet M-500 Vitamins) each day. Alcohol poisons liver cells that may already be on the critical list, and alcoholic beverages should be shunned as you would a social disease. Whiskey, beer, wine and all other alcohol-containing beverages are forbidden; replace them with milk, water, coffee, tea, and fruit juices.

With the better-diet, no-alcohol self-help treatment described plus medical therapy prescribed by his physician, the individual with incipient cirrhosis can expect to improve the function of his liver and hopefully to avoid the ominous complications of advanced cirrhosis.

COLITIS

Synonyms: spastic colitis, irritable bowel

In the nineteenth century, Josh Billings (Henry Wheeler Shaw) wrote, "I have finally kum to the konklusion, that a good reliable sett ov bowels iz wurth more tu a man, than enny quantity ov brains." The alternative is a troublesome colon, manifested as diarrhea, constipation, cramps, or any combination of these three. The disease, as a rule, is chronic, with colitis symptoms recurring whenever the victim suffers an emotional upheaval or is guilty of a dietary indiscretion.

Taming the Irritable Colon

Diet plays a decisive role in overcoming an irritable bowel. Avoid spicy foods, as well as excessively hot and cold foods.

No coffee, tea, or alcohol is permitted, since these may aggravate an irritable bowel.

A recent medical study has shown the value of unprocessed bran and a high-fiber diet in the treatment of the irritable bowel syndrome. Fiber—sometimes called roughage—is the food component that is not digested but remains in the intestinal tract to absorb water and form the bulk of solid waste. A diet high in plant fiber helps intestinal movement in constipation-prone patients, while individuals with diarrhea showed a relaxation of bowel overactivity. When fed to normal individuals without bowel symptoms, the diet generally causes no change in bowel motility.

Eat at least five grams of fiber daily, which requires six to eight servings of fruits, vegetables, whole grain breads and cereals, plus other high-fiber foods. Plant fiber can be added to the diet as bran flakes taken in the morning, or perhaps as a rounded teaspoonful of powdered psyllium hydrophilic mucilloid (Metamucil) taken at bedtime. Since some fiber, such as that in seeds, provides bulk, while other fiber, such as in apples, absorbs water, it's best to get your daily fiber intake from a variety of foods.

The following chart can be a guide in selecting your high-fiber diet:

High-Fiber Diet

	gm fiber		gm fiber
Main Dishes (1 cup)			
Beans and franks	2.6	Chili con carne	1.8
Beans with pork	1.6	Chow mein	1.1
Beef stew	1.2		
Beans & Legumes			
(1 cup)			
Baked beans with pork and		Lentils, cooked	2.2
tomato sauce	3.6	Lima beans, cooked	2.9
Black beans, cooked	3.0	Pinto beans, cooked	2.3
Chickpeas, cooked	2.5	Split peas, cooked	1.0
Kidney beans, cooked	2.3	White beans, cooked	2.2

	gm fiber		gm fiber

Vegetables
(½ cup, or as noted)

	gm fiber		gm fiber
Beans, green	.6	Okra, sliced	.8
Beet greens	1.1	Onion (2½")	.6
Beets, diced	.7	chopped raw	.6
Broccoli	1.1	Peas	1.6
Brussels sprouts	1.1	Peppers, sweet	1.0
Carrots, 1 medium	.8	Potato, baked, 1 medium	.7
diced	.6	Rutabagas	1.1
Cauliflower	.6	Sauerkraut	.9
Coleslaw	.8	Spinach	.6
Corn, kernels	.7	Squash, acorn	1.6
cream	.6	Sweet potato, 1 small	1.0
Cucumber, 1 medium	1.7	Tomato, 1 medium	.8
pared	.6	Turnip greens	.7
Eggplant, pared and diced	.9	Turnips	.6
Mushrooms, canned	.6		

Fruits
(½ cup, or as noted)

	gm fiber		gm fiber
Apple, 1 medium	1.5	Orange, 1 medium	.8
Applesauce, canned	.7	Peach, raw, 1 medium	.6
Avocado, 4 oz.	1.6	Pears, canned, 2 halves	.6
Banana, 1 medium	.8	raw, 1 medium	2.8
Blackberries	3.0	Prunes, pitted	1.2
Blueberries	1.1	Raspberries	
Cantaloupe, ½ medium	.6	black	3.8
Dates, pitted	2.1	red	2.0
Honeydew, 2" x 7" wedge	.9	Strawberries	1.0

Breads, Cereals, Pasta, Rice

	gm fiber		gm fiber
Cereals, 1 ounce		Macaroni, dry, 8 oz.	.7
All-Bran	2.1	Bran muffins (3")	.7
Bran Buds	2.0	Noodles, dry, 8 oz.	.7
Bran Flakes	1.0	Rice, brown, dry	
40% Bran Flakes	1.0	½ cup	.8
Raisin Bran	.9	Whole wheat roll	
Wheat Chex	.8	1 medium	.6
Corn meal, dry, 1 cup	.8	Spaghetti, dry, 8 oz.	.7
Whole wheat flour	2.8		

Medication is often prescribed by the doctor if the irritable bowel syndrome fails to respond to diet therapy. The products prescribed are intended to allay cramps and reduce bowel overactivity; common choices include mepenzolate bromide (Cantil), dicyclomine hydrochloride (Bentyl), or methixene hydrochloride (Trest). Anxiety associated with bowel irritability may be treated with Donnatal or Librax— both containing a mild tranquilizer in addition to a spasmtaming ingredient.

If severe diarrhea occurs, the choice may be over-the-counter Donnagel containing kaolin and pectin, plus a belladonna-like medication to reduce bowel spasm; but for severe diarrhea, the physician often prescribes diphenoxylate hydrochloride with atropine (Lomotil). When diarrhea is acute, one good remedy is small quantities of skimmed milk heated just to a boil, then cooled. Six to eight ounces three times daily is about right, sipped slowly or taken with a spoon.

Avoiding Bowel Problems

Many symptoms of the irritable colon can be avoided through proper bowel hygiene. This means eating plenty of fresh fruit, vegetables, and whole grain products, consuming lots of fluids, and exercising regularly. The urge to defecate should be heeded promptly, and harsh laxatives should be avoided. Finally, any change in bowel function, particularly if bleeding is involved, should be checked by the physician.

CONJUNCTIVITIS

Synonyms: pinkeye, eye infection

Conjunctivitis is an irritation or infection of the outer surface of the eye, and usually involves the inner lining of the eyelids. The white of the eye is red and irritated, and there is an uncomfortable scratchy sensation. If infection is present, droplets of pus may be noted, although conjunctivitis is often caused by viruses (which do not form pus) or by irritation due to fumes, chlorine, or allergy.

Treatment

Mildly irritated eyes can often be treated safely at home.

Don't rub, since this intensifies the irritation and contaminated fingertips may spread infection to the other eye. Avoid dust, fumes, and tobacco smoke that may contribute to conjunctival inflammation. Troublesome sources of allergy should be avoided whenever possible, including animal dander, grass or tree pollens, ragweed pollen, and house dust.

Eye irritation usually responds to simple decongestant eye drops. A well-advertised and highly effective preparation is Visine Eye Drops, whose active ingredient is tetrahydrozoline hydrochloride. Two drops of Visine in each irritated eye helps "get the red out," and may be repeated three or four times daily. Another effective over-the-counter preparation is Ey-Gene Ophthalmic Solution, containing the decongestant phenylephrine hydrochloride, together with peppermint water, thimerosal, boric acid, borax, salt, sodium bisulfate, and camphor water.

Infectious conjunctivitis due to viral organisms or pus-forming bacteria may respond to preparations containing zinc sulfate. Two such preparations, both containing zinc sulfate along with the decongestant phenylephrine hydrochloride, are Zincfrin Eye Drops and Prince Matchabelli Aziza Medicated Eye Drops. Two drops in each eye every two to four hours help relieve irritating conjunctival congestion and combat bacterial infection.

The Red Eye Problem

Not all red eyes are caused by conjunctivitis. Other possible causes include iritis (which often impairs vision) or glaucoma (which may cause a deep aching discomfort). And to further confuse the diagnosis, many cases of conjunctivitis fail to respond to the remedies listed above.

Therefore, here are the guidelines. If eye irritation appears minor and scratchy, if there is no deep aching pain, and no distortion of vision, it is usually safe to self-treat minor eye irritations with the preparations discussed above—for up to 48 hours.

However, if the irritation seems especially severe, if deep pain is present, or if there is any visual distortion, however slight, see the physician without delay.

CONSTIPATION

Synonym: sluggish bowel

Most persons who think they are constipated really aren't. There's a popular misconception, carefully nurtured by laxative manufacturers, that a daily bowel movement is essential to good health. It isn't, and a bowel movement every third or fourth day is no more or less healthy than the daily always-after-breakfast evacuation.

In fact, the one-a-day bowel movement fantasy can be harmful as individuals consume ever-increasing quantities of laxatives to achieve their ideal. In time, the bowel can become laxative-dependent, and normal unassisted evacuation ceases.

Avoiding Constipation

Constipation is prevented and treated by careful attention to proper bowel habits.

Bowel hygiene sets the stage: Fluids are essential to prevent dried-out feces from forming in the rectum. Exercise stimulates peristaltic activity, and a brisk walk once or twice daily can help keep the bowels moving. Refined carbohydrates impair bowel movement while the addition of bran and plant fibers to the diet can help normalize bowel function (see the high-fiber diet on page 72). Finally, when the urge to evacuate is felt, heed it promptly; if you don't respond, tardiness may cause the urge to disappear.

Diet therapy for constipation calls for a liberal intake of high-roughage foods, including vegetables and fruits, whole grain cereals and breads; plus fluids of all kinds such as water, juices, buttermilk, etc. In my professional experience the following diet has helped control constipation.

Specific recommendations include a morning glass of prune juice, a bowl of bran cereal, and an increased intake of high-fiber foods such as celery, beans, lettuce, cabbage, rhubarb, spinach, and carrots.

Foods Permitted	*Foods to Be Avoided*

Cereals

Take 2 tablespoonfuls of natural unprocessed bran daily	Sugar-coated cereals
Cooked oat and wheat cereals	
Dry precooked cereals	
Bran cereals	

Breads

Whole wheat bread	White bread
Corn bread	Rolls and biscuits made with refined flour
Pancakes and waffles	
Bran muffins	

Soups

Creamed soups	Bouillon and broth
Meat stock soups	
Bean, lentil, or split pea soups	

Meat, Fish, and Dairy Products

Boiled, baked, or broiled veal, ham, lean beef, turkey or chicken, and fish	Mutton and pork
Shellfish	Fried or fatty meats
Soft cooked eggs	Fried eggs
Cheese	
Cottage Cheese	

Vegetables

Cucumbers	Pureed vegetables
Carrots	Onions
Brussels sprouts	Radishes
Lettuce	
Turnips	
Peas	
Potatoes	
Spinach	
Tomatoes	
Corn	
Cabbage	
Beets	
Celery	
Asparagus	
Green beans	
Squash	

Foods Permitted	Foods to Be Avoided

Fruits

All raw fruits	Pureed fruits
Cooked fruits	
Fruit juices	
Rhubarb	

Deserts

Sherbet	Cakes
Gelatin	Pies and pastries
Fruit ice	Custard and pudding
Apricot whip	Ice cream
Prune whip	Bread pudding
	Tapioca pudding
	Rice pudding

Beverages

Drink 6 glasses of water daily, between meals and at bedtime	Alcoholic beverages
	Whole milk
Coffee, tea	
Decaffeinated coffee	
Carbonated beverages	
Cocoa, Postum, and Ovaltine	
Skimmed milk	
Buttermilk	

Miscellaneous

Liquid vegetable oils (corn, soybean, and safflower)	Animal fats and lard
	Macaroni and spaghetti
Sugar	Mayonnaise
Salt	Gravy
Pepper	Candy
Olives	
Pickles	
Tomato paste	
Garlic	
Mustard	
Horseradish	
Jelly and Jam	
Relish	
Vinegar	
Honey and molasses	

Proper bowel hygiene and dietary diligence notwithstanding, the colon occasionally needs a little help. Sometimes it's a gentle push; for other individuals medication may be a daily ritual. Most products to combat constipation need no prescription, but it's important to understand the advantages and limitations of any medication used.

Rectal suppositories aid evacuation of a reluctant rectum. The standard is the glycerin suppository, causing evacuation as it stimulates rectal tissues and helps soften feces. More potent is the bisacodyl (Dulcolax) 10-mg rectal suppository, usually promoting bowel evacuation within one hour after insertion.

Enemas, like suppositories, ease the evacuation of feces languishing in the colon and rectum. For generations, hospital nurses have used a frothy mixture of warm soapsuds prepared from hospital green soap and tap water. Today, the most widely used enema preparation is the disposable Fleet Enema containing sodium phosphate and biphosphate. Sold in a disposable plastic bottle with an applicator tip, the Fleet Enema usually empties the colon within a few minutes after administration.

Stool softeners, sometimes called lubricant laxatives, aid evacuation by moving feces smoothly through the bowel. The prototype product is mineral oil, now known to be hazardous in long-term use; prolonged administration can interfere with the absorption of fat-soluble Vitamins A, D, K, and E. The modern product is dioctyl sodium sulfosuccinate (Colace) taken in a usual adult dosage of a single 100-mg tablet daily.

The bulk-forming laxatives modify the stool's consistency—softening, smoothing, and promoting effortless evacuation without the spasm of harsher laxatives. Like dioctyl sulfosuccinate, the bulk-formers can be used daily to promote regular evacuation. One widely used product is hydrophylic mucilloid of psyllium (Metamucil), available as a powder (one teaspoonful in one glass of water taken at bedtime) or as Metamucil instant mix (an effervescent powder; pour the contents of one packet into one glass of water and drink as soon as dissolved).

The saline cathartics are more potent. Various salts are poorly absorbed by the body from the intestine. These draw water into the bowel, adding fluid to the feces and stimulating the muscular contraction that speeds the waste matter toward its destination. Citrate of magnesia is a time-honored favorite, as is magnesium hydroxide suspension (milk of magnesia). A potent preparation in this group is sodium biphosphate and phosphate (Fleet's Phospho-Soda).

The stimulant cathartics are irritating laxatives that spur the tired bowel into activity. These harsh laxatives should be used sparingly, if at all, and daily administration can soon result in laxative dependence. Castor oil and cascara are potent prototypes of this group. Senna products have an irritant action not unlike cascara, and usually produce evacuation within six hours: The Senokot brand of senna products is widely sold, and less-well-known senna-containing cathartics include Black Draught Syrup (containing senna and rhubarb), Innerclean Granules (containing senna, fragula, psyllium, and agar), and Gentlax Granules (containing senna and guar gum). Phenolphthalein laxatives include Ex-Lax (containing yellow phenolphthalein), Agoral (containing phenolphthalein and mineral oil), Correctol (containing yellow phenolphthalein and dioctyl sodium sufosuccinate), and Feen-a-Mint gum tablets (containing yellow phenolphthalein).

Laxatives aren't harmless just because they can be purchased without prescription. Administration of a stimulant cathartic to a patient with abdominal pain and vomiting could cause rupture of the bowel. Like most other medications in the pharmacy, skillful administration can bring blessed relief of symptoms, while uninformed use may be hazardous.

CONTACT RASH

Synonym: contact dermatitis

When susceptible skin comes in contact with poison ivy, nickel, kerosene products, or a host of other allergens, contact dermatitis results. Poison ivy is the prototype, and most individuals suffer (or have the potential for) sensitivity to the resin of the poison ivy plant. Ubiquitous nickel—found in coins, jewelry, eyeglass frames, zippers, fasteners, and hundreds of other inconspicuous artifacts—is a common cause of contact rashes, as are many other items, including detergents, dyes, perfumes, solutions used to tan leather, woolens, airborne pollens that settle on clothing, synthetic fabrics, cosmetics, local anesthetics, and preservatives in skin preparations including those the doctor may prescribe.

On the skin, the rash appears the same—red, blistered, and intensely itching—regardless of the cause. But the location may give a clue: poison ivy strikes the exposed areas of the hands, wrists, and face; a nickel allergy may be limited to the skin under a metal watchband or the earlobes following wearing of earrings containing nickel; a red rash of the wrists and neck may occur where an offending perfume was dabbed.

But often the cause is obscure, and detective work is needed to nail the culprit. I saw one patient, for instance, with four dots of contact dermatitis on the right cheek, occurring as she leaned her chin on her hand and resulting from sensitivity to her nail polish. Another patient had a perfect rectangle outlined on his left thigh; the cause was a leaking old-fashioned flip-top cigarette lighter, with the image of the lighter traced on the leg as a lighter-fluid allergic reaction.

What to Do about the Contact Rash?

Avoid the allergenic cause whenever possible; that's the easy way to prevent contact dermatitis. The poison ivy-sensitive individual must garden only with gloved hands and avoid barelegged woodland strolls. The nickel-allergic individual can wear only pure gold jewelry. And the cosmetic-sensitive woman should use no makeup or perhaps switch to the hypoallergenic brands such as Almay or Allercreme.

A blistered, draining contact rash must be dried before creams or ointments are applied. Moist compresses dry oozing skin rashes, and a useful household soak is one teaspoonful of table salt dissolved in a pint of warm water, applied as a moist compress for 30 minutes four or five times daily. Remember how salt water dried your skin at the beach last summer? A saline soak achieves the same result. Even more effective (but involving a trip to the pharmacy) is a Burow's solution soak made with Domeboro Powder Packets. Dissolve one powder packet in a pint of warm water and use as a soak for one-half hour four times daily.

As the draining area dries, healing may be aided by old-fashioned Calamine Lotion. More sophisticated is Surfadil

Lotion containing the antihistamine methapyrilene hydrochloride, the local anesthetic cyclomethycaine, and the drying agent titanium dioxide.

Dry contact dermatitis lesions are best treated with creams and lotions. Reasonable choices include Acid Mantle Cream containing aluminum acetate, or Lubriderm Lotion containing oxycholesterin, sorbitol, mineral oil, triethanolamine stearate, cetyl alcohol, and paraben esters. Infinitely more effective are the cortisone creams, lotions, and ointments, such as generic ¼-percent hydrocortisone cream, betamethasone (Valisone) cream, or fluocinonide (Lidex) cream.

Cortisone by pills or injection may be prescribed for acute contact dermatitis, particularly when widespread poison ivy-induced swelling threatens to close the eyes and swell the hands into immobility.

Poison ivy extract injections (Ivyol) are available to provide modest protection against poison ivy dermatitis, but the best defense against this and all other types of contact rash is arm's-lengh avoidance of the causative substance.

CONTRACEPTION

Synonym: birth control

Reliable contraception is one of the joys of modern civilization, allowing husband and wife to plan the size of their family rather than simply accepting offspring when and if they "occur." Many methods are available, some more reliable than others, although with each increase in efficacy comes a corresponding rise in potential side effects.

The following is a survey of contraceptive methods currently available.

The Rhythm Method

The premise of the rhythm method of contraception is this: Approximately 14 days after the onset of the menstrual period an egg is released by the ovary. The release of the egg is called ovulation, and may be signaled by a slight discomfort on one side of the pelvis. The released egg promptly enters the Fallopian tube and it is here that fertilization may take place. The rhythm method aims to identify the time of ovulation and avoid sexual intercourse during this danger period.

The woman with a more-or-less regular menstrual cycle usually ovulates about day 14 and simple counting helps identify the danger time. Sexual relations can be enjoyed with relative safety up to three days before and beginning three days after the presumed time of ovulation.

More scientific is measurement of the basal body temperature to detect the time of ovulation. Ovulation is marked by a brief fall, then sustained slight elevation, in body temperature. The higher temperature following ovulation persists until just before the menstrual flow, but is of such small magnitude (about 0.5 degree Fahrenheit) that utmost care must be exercised in reporting the daily temperature. A rectal thermometer is more accurate than an oral temperature determination and a special "Cycletemp" thermometer is recommended. The temperature is taken each morning at the time of awakening before arising from bed, eating, or drinking. The resulting daily graph will help pinpoint the day of ovulation and aid in the timing of sexual relations.

A word of caution is in order: Despite careful counting and apparently precise basal body temperature determinations, pregnancy occasionally occurs on day 8 or day 10 or day 19, and rhythm method contraception is recommended only for those couples who wouldn't mind raising a large family.

Condom

The condom, or "rubber," will prevent most pregnancies. It is inexpensive, easily available, but is spurned by many males as clumsy and impairing sensitivity. This objection has been partially overcome by current models, which are thinner than in the past, and some condoms today have surface ridges reported to increase sexual satisfaction.

The condom has the advantage of helping prevent the spread of venereal disease and should be used whenever the possibility of infection is present.

Vaginal Foams and Creams

Vaginal creams, jellies, and aerosol foams are often used to form a chemical and mechanical barrier to contraception.

Current evidence suggests that aerosol foams may be more effective than creams and jellies while suppositories are considered least effective since they must melt in the vagina before becoming active. The relatively large bulk of aerosol foam seems reponsible for its greater effectiveness. Messiness is a drawback and occasionally one or both sexual partners develop irritation due to chemical constituents of the preparation. Reliable products are Delfen Cream and Foam (Delfen Foam reports a 99% success rate when used regularly), and Preceptin Contraceptive Gel.

Diaphragm and Jelly

Until the development of birth control pills, the diaphragm and jelly served as the leading contraceptive method of most married couples. When oral contraceptives became popular twelve to fifteen years ago, diaphragm use dropped dramatically. However, during the past few years many women have become anxious concerning possible side effects of oral contraceptives and intrauterine devices, and the diaphragm is once again finding favor as a contraceptive device.

Consisting of a flexible ring supporting a rubber dome, the diaphragm must be carefully fitted by a physician and inserted dexterously so that the cervix (mouth of the womb) is covered. Addition of a contraceptive jelly such as Ortho-Gynol Contraceptive Jelly to the dome of the diaphragm aids effectiveness and is an integral part of the technique. The diaphragm must, of course, be inserted prior to sexual relations and is left in place for eight hours following sexual union.

I recall one gynecologist who counseled his patients that "diaphragm and jelly are 100% effective if used correctly." The occasional failure was easily explained: "You used it incorrectly."

Oral Contraceptives

Ease, simplicity, and virtual hundred-percent effectiveness have made birth control pills the leading contraceptive method in America today. When "the pill" is used properly, fewer than one woman out of one hundred will become pregnant and oral contraceptives are the method of choice for most young women who would find a diaphragm cumbersome and whose uterus might not tolerate an intrauterine device. Oral contraceptives produce light periods with minimal cramps but an increased likelihood of candidal vaginal infections.

With millions of women taking this medication daily, much attention has focused upon side effects. Blood clots in the legs are a known hazard and medical studies reveal an increased risk of 3 per 100,000 cases. In addition, 1976 studies have linked birth control pills with heart attacks, primarily in women over age 40. In general, the risk of dangerous side effects is less in younger women taking lower dose pills and greater in older women taking oral contraceptives with a higher estrogen content. As with all medication for long-term use, the benefits of oral contraception must be weighed against the possibility of side effects and the physician should be consulted for his advice.

Intrauterine Device

Many women concerned about the long-term use of birth control pills have turned to the intrauterine device and the IUD is finding increased favor with young women who have never borne children. The concept of the IUD originated many centuries ago when camel drivers inserted stones into the wombs of their female camels to prevent pregnancy on long desert journeys. Intrauterine contraceptive devices for human use caught on in Europe in the 1950s with the Graefenberg ring, followed by the Margolis coil, then the Lippes loope and the Dalkon shield. Currently popular contraceptive devices include the Copper 7 and Copper T (which use the chemical properties of copper) and the new Progestasert Therapeutic System which releases small doses of the hormone progesterone within the uterus. All IUDs may cause bleeding and cramps, most noticeable during the first few months.

Surgical Sterilization

Surgical contraception, including vasectomy in the male and ligation of the female Fallopian tubes, affords permanent contraception, but necessitates a surgical procedure. Vasectomy is usually performed in the doctor's office or hospital outpatient department. The procedure is brief, only local anesthesia is needed, and most patients return to work the next day.

Laproscopic techniques have made possible surgical sterilization of the female by ligation of the Fallopian tubes. A tiny incision is made in the abdominal wall or vagina and surgery is performed through a telescope-like instrument. Complications are few and postoperative discomfort is minimal.

Surgical sterilization is not for the faint of heart; there is no turning back and efforts to reverse surgical contraception are rarely fruitful.

On the Horizon

Spurred by the ready market for reliable contraceptive methods, doctors and pharmaceutical manufacturers continue to experiment with new methods, including an injectable agent for females, injectable or oral agents for males, an open-and-shut vasectomy valve, vaginal rings, and even chemical compounds to induce early abortions. But general use of these methods is probably years away.

CONVULSIONS

Synonyms: convulsive seizures, epilepsy

There is much confusion about convulsions. Here are the quick facts you need to know for self-help prevention and care of convulsive seizures.

A convulsion begins with a nerve discharge in the brain, much like a short circuit in a fuse box. The sparks set off electrical impulses in the nerve, affecting consciousness and body movements according to the location of the disturbance in the brain.

Seizures have many causes. A rising temperature in a susceptible infant can cause the febrile convulsion. Sometimes seizures are caused by scar tissue from an old injury. Brain damage at birth may be the cause; occasionally a cancerous growth is the culprit, although most convulsive seizures are of unknown cause.

The Types of Seizures

Contributing to the misconceptions about seizures are the many types of convulsions found:

- Grand mal epilepsy is the classic convulsive seizure, beginning suddenly with the patient showing jerking movements of all extremities, chewing movements of the teeth (which may injure the tongue), and arching of the neck. Before long, the jerking subsides and the patient suffers an overwhelming tiredness. The prescribed drug treatment for grand mal epilepsy may include phenobarbital (in use as an anticonvulsive medicine since 1912), diphenylhydantoin (Dilantin), primidone (Mysoline), or carbamazepine (Tegretol).
- Petit mal, also called absence seizures, is a sudden loss of awareness, usually seen as an unresponsive blank stare. Most episodes last about 10 seconds, perhaps less, and there may be movements of the hands or head. Petit mal seizures may occur infrequently or perhaps dozens of times a day. Drug treatment often includes one or more of the following: ethosuximide (Zarontin), methsuximide (Celontin), phensuximide (Milontin), or trimethadone (Tridione).
- Psychomotor seizures are sometimes called temporal lobe seizures indicating their site of origin in the brain. These complex attacks may cause a wide spectrum of manifestations, including sudden fright, chewing movements, running, or garbled speech. Following the attack there is amnesia concerning the episode, although an occasional individual recalls fragments as though from a dream. Often linked with grand mal seizures, psychomotor seizures may herald the onset of a major convulsive attack. Drugs often prescribed include diphenylhydantoin (Dilantin), phenobarbital, primidone (Mysoline), and carbamazepine (Tegretol).
- Febrile convulsions occur in at least 2 percent of all children, and are usually seen between the ages of six months and four years. It's important to know that children known to suffer febrile seizures will often convulse as the fever passes 102°F, while the otherwise normal child usually will not convulse even with a fever above 105°F. Elixir phenobarbital taken by

mouth helps prevent recurrences of seizures. When I encounter a youngster known to be susceptible to febrile convulsions, I recommend that phenobarbital administration begin at the first sign of any illness that might cause fever. At some time following age four, the use of phenobarbital can be stopped.

- Minor motor seizures are a disorder of youngsters up to age three years. The child gives a series of sudden jerks, perhaps lasting for several minutes, and then there are no symptoms until the attack recurs. Minor motor seizures are poorly controlled with medication, although some respond to cortisone treatment. The jerking attacks usually cease by the fourth birthday, although many youngsters are left with mental impairment.

Self-Help Advice for Seizures

From reading the above, it's clear that convlusive seizures are complex and require professional advice. In fact, most family physicians refer their seizure patients for neurological consultation. Self-help treatment aims to supplement the doctor's advice and medication. Here are basic principles:

- Convulsive seizures may be brought on by flashing lights, and sometimes occur with susceptible youngsters watching a flickering television set. If you have a seizure-prone child, be careful to monitor his TV viewing.
- Febrile convulsions are abnormal reactions to fever. An important aspect of emergency self-help treatment is lowering the temperature. Remove all clothing from the infant, and sponge him with water a little cooler than room temperature, allowing evaporation to cool the body.
- The grand mal seizure will almost always subside, regardless of the treatment. Prevent the victim from injury due to falling or crashing into nearby objects. If there are chewing movements, place a firm yet pliable object between the teeth; a man's belt is just right. Never place your finger between the gnashing teeth of an epileptic or the physician will have two patients instead of one. Loosen tight clothing and turn the head

to one side so that secretions or vomit will not be inhaled. Take a good look because later someone may ask you to describe the seizure; then send for an ambulance.

- Restrain the urge to overtreat the epileptic. Brandy or coffee poured down his throat may go into the lungs instead. Ill-advised attempts to move him may cause injury. When a convulsion occurs, it's an emergency where it may be best to do less, and hasty action can cause great harm.

- The seizure-prone individual must never, never stop his pills abruptly, even if in the hospital for other reasons. The penalty for abrupt drug cessation may be status epilepticus—a recurring series of epileptic attacks that sometimes defies treatment and may end fatally.

For the afflicted individual and his family, there's much to be learned about convulsive seizures. Here are three sources of information:

Epilepsy Foundation of America
1828 L Street, N.W.
Washington, D.C. 20036

American Epilepsy Foundation
77 Reservoir Road
Quincy, Massachusetts 02167

National Epilepsy League
203 North Wabash Avenue
Chicago, Illinois 60610

CROUP

Synonyms: laryngotracheobronchitis, tracheobronchitis

Caring for the child with croup gives mothers—and doctors—gray hair. The croupy cough, a high-pitched bark that sounds like a seal at the zoo, signals partial closure of the airway and strikes terror in the hearts of those hearing it for the first time. Doctors appreciate the dangers of croup, and physicians who may say "ho-hum" to flu or the common cold will leap from bed to attend a youngster with croup.

Croup describes an irritation and swelling of the membranes of the respiratory passages, occurring when a susceptible child suffers a cold, and it often is linked with a change in the weather such as the onset of a storm. When I see a croup patient in my family practice office in the morning, I expect to see more croup or asthma victims later that day—or, more likely, in the wee hours of the morning when croup is usually at its worst.

Coping with Croup

Step one in caring for the croupy child is a call to the physician. His advice is vital; he may be needed in an emergency after midnight, and it's only fair to allow him to participate in the early care of the disease. He will almost certainly recommend a cold-steam vaporizer—in the child's room at night, moved with him about the house during the day. Inhaling vapor helps dissolve sticky phlegm that is blocking the airway, and acute shortness of breath can sometimes be alleviated by sitting in a steam-filled bathroom as a running warm shower fills the room with vapor. Drinking fluids helps dissolve dried-out secretions; that's why doctors usually advise patients with colds to "take plenty of fluids."

Thick secretions can be cleared using an expectorant cough mixture. Unless the cough is incapacitating, it's often best to avoid cough suppressants such as codeine or dextromethorphan. A first-rate prescription expectorant cough medicine is Robitussin, containing glyceryl guaiacolate, taken in a dose of one teaspoon every four to six hours depending upon the patient's age and weight.

Since croup seems to be the first cousin of asthma, preparations used against asthma may be helpful in the treatment of laryngotracheobronchitis. One such product is Tedral Elixir containing theophylline to open tight bronchial airways, the decongestant ephedrine, and phenobarbital for sedation, all in a 15-percent alcohol base. Tedral Expectorant contains the above ingredients plus glyceryl guaiacolate to dissolve mucus.

Aspirin is given as needed for fever. The dose should be one grain of aspirin per year of age (to a maximum 10-grain dose), taken every six to eight hours if fever is present.

The physician will prescribe an appropriate antibiotic if bacterial infection is present, and occasionally epinephrine or cortisone will be administered if severe airway spasm is present. Many youngsters with croup require hospitalization for intensive therapy, which may include a "croup tent" or even a tracheotomy to ensure adequate breathing. Because of the potential seriousness of the disease, croup treatment should always be undertaken with the advice of your physician.

CYSTIC FIBROSIS

Synonyms: CF, cystic fibrosis of the pancreas

One baby in approximately every 2,000 is born with this genetic disorder, which attacks Caucasians almost exclusively. Only 5 percent of those affected live past the age of 17.

In cystic fibrosis, thick mucus plugs the bronchial tubes, causing respiratory infections, and blocks the pancreatic ducts, impairing digestion and causing malnutrition. Common symptoms are frequent coughing, rapid breathing, diarrhea, failure of a baby to gain weight despite excellent appetite, and sweat with a very high salt content (often allowing the alert mother to suspect the diagnosis as her infant tastes salty when kissed). For information write to:

National Cystic Fibrosis Research Foundation
Suite 950
3379 Peachtree Road, N.E.
Atlanta, Georgia 30326

DANDRUFF

Synonym: seborrhea of the scalp

An advertisement once said, "Don't blame your hair for what your scalp is doing to your head." Dandruff is a scalp disease, with hair an innocent victim caught in the struggle between an oily scalp and therapeutic shampoo preparations.

Doctors call dandruff seborrhea of the scalp, and the medical term seborrhea comes from two Greek words meaning "to flow with fat." Although the flakes of dandruff seem dry, the disorder is one of superabundant scalp secretions drying to form dandruff flakes. Dandruff, like acne (another disorder caused by oily secretions), is common during the teen-age years and often strikes dark complexions more savagely than light. With age, skin and scalp secretions dwindle and dandruff often becomes less troublesome. But, in the meantime . . .

Defeating Dandruff

The key to conquering dandruff is removal of scalp oils. Keep in mind that there is no cure. Dandruff can be controlled by regular removal of excessive secretions, but a lapse in treatment will be followed by scaling flakes fluttering from the scalp. While it helps to minimize the intake of high-fat greasy foods such as potato chips, deep-fried delicacies, and fatty cuts of meat, the cornerstone of dandruff therapy remains the therapeutic shampoo.

Antidandruff shampoos are available from many manufacturers. Common ingredients include selenium sulfide (probably our most potent antidandruff remedy), tar derivatives, flake-softening salicylic acid, and detergents. Here is a list of useful preparations available without prescription:

- Head and Shoulders Dandruff Shampoo contains zinc pyrithione. Creative advertising has made it a sales leader and it's a worthwhile preparation, although not the strongest on the market.
- Meted Anti-Dandruff Shampoo contains sulfur, salicylic acid, and triclocarban. It's a reliable preparation when used according to package directions.
- Sebulex Antiseborrheic Shampoo contains sulfur, salicylic acid, and cleansers. I have recommended this product for years as a remedy for infant cradle cap, which is after all merely dandruff of the baby's scalp.
- Selsun Blue Shampoo, containing 1 percent selenium sulfide is, in my opinion, the most potent over-the-counter dandruff remedy. Some individuals require its use once or twice weekly. The manufacturer recommends that if used before or after tinting, bleaching, or permanent waving, the hair should be rinsed for at least five minutes in cool running water. Also avail-

able by prescription is Selsun Lotion (2½ percent selenium sulfide for superstubborn dandruff.

DEAFNESS

Synonym: impaired hearing

Sound waves enter the auditory apparatus (see Figure 9) through the ear canal and cause vibrations of the eardrum (tympanic membrane), which in turn sets in motion the three small bones of the middle ear—the hammer, anvil, and stirrup. The stirrup (stapes) passes the vibration to the inner ear, from which the auditory nerve carries impulses to the brain.

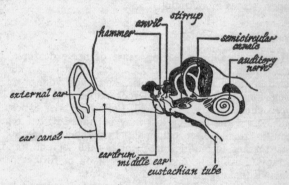

FIGURE 9. *The normal ear.*

Hearing loss may follow damage to the conduction mechanism, including ear canal, eardrum, or middle ear bones, while other individuals suffer nerve (perception) deafness caused by damage to the auditory nerve or brain hearing center.

Conduction Deafness

Wax in the ear canal is a common and easily treatable cause of hearing loss. The onset is often somewhat abrupt, with reduced hearing and a sense of pressure in the ear canal. Local applications of carbamide, peroxide, and anhydrous glycerol (Debrox) drops may remove stubborn ear wax, or at least soften the plug to facilitate removal by the physician.

Middle ear infections gum up the hearing mechanism, including eardrum and small middle ear bones. A common cause of childhood hearing loss, middle ear infections may respond to antibiotic and decongestant therapy, but sometimes require surgery with incision of the eardrum (myringotomy) and perhaps the insertion of a tube into the tympanic membrane to aid drainage.

A chronically scarred or perforated eardrum may hamper hearing or cause no defect at all. If hearing loss is present, the doctor may repair the eardrum.

A conduction hearing loss may follow stiffness of the stirrup (stapes) as it communicates with the inner ear, and hearing may return dramatically following surgery to free the stapes (stapes mobilization).

Nerve Deafness

Loud noises are a leading cause of nerve deafness, common among artillery veterans, hunters, industrial workers subjected to loud machinery noise, and even youngsters who spend long hours listening to rock music with decibel levels approaching the pain threshold. Following brief exposure to loud noises, the hearing loss may be transient; but repeated acoustic trauma often culminates in permanent hearing loss, most marked in the high frequencies—the soprano tones. No therapy is available, and the preservation of further hearing demands that exposure to loud noises cease.

There also is no effective treatment for congenital nerve deafness (hereditary deafness) or for the nerve deafness that occurs with aging.

Some drugs can cause impaired hearing, and these include streptomycin, kanamycin, vancomycin, neomycin, ethacrynic acid, and quinine. If auditory involvement is suspected, the drug is stopped immediately, and the hearing may or may not return.

Less common causes of nerve deafness include intracranial tumors, syphilis, and encephalitis. Early treatment of these diseases may spare hearing.

Hold on to Your Hearing

Here are some simple self-help rules to preserve hearing:

- Don't probe the ear with applicator sticks, hairpins, or other foreign objects. The ear cleans itself efficiently, and manipulation can have dire consequences.
- Avoid exposure to loud noises, and use ear plugs or shields if you must be in an area where loud sounds occur.
- Try not to fly in an airplane or dive deep in a swimming pool if you have a common cold. Sudden pressure changes in the presence of a respiratory infection can cause middle ear disease.
- Be sure young girls receive the rubella (German measles) vaccine, which affords lifelong protection; congenital deafness is one of the consequences of rubella contracted by the mother-to-be.
- Avoid drugs that can cause hearing loss.
- Suspect a hearing impairment if an infant fails to respond to sound or the spoken word or if his speech development is slow.
- See your physician if you suspect hearing loss, since many causes are treatable.
- Don't buy a hearing aid without a consultation with an otologist.

For further information about hearing loss, write to:

National Association of Hearing and Speech Agencies
919 18th Street, N.W.
Washington, D.C. 20006

DEPRESSION

Synonyms: mental depression, psychic depression

They call depression the common cold of mental illnesses. It's as common as crabgrass and as dispiriting as a rainy weekend, for it blights the outlook and dampens all enthusiasm. Symptoms of depression include lethargy, poor appetite, and lack of interest in getting a job done. There's fatigue all day, difficulty falling asleep at night, then awakening early in the morning unable to doze again.

Depression is not only as common as the cold but, like this ubiquitous viral infection, can have serious complications. Up to eight million Americans suffer depression each year and a quarter million require hospitalization—for active treatment and as prophylaxis against suicide. Not only the common man or woman suffers depression; the disease pervades all levels of society. Thomas Eagleton's chances for the Vice Presidency were shattered in 1972 when the public found out about his previous hospitalizations for depression. Winston Churchill took up painting to relieve his anxious depressions. Depression drove Ernest Hemingway to suicide, and friends of Abraham Lincoln feared a self-destructive act when he wrote in 1841: "If what I feel were equally distributed to the whole human family, there would not be one cheerful face on earth."

Overcoming Depression

Learn to recognize the symptoms of depression: gradual deterioration from a well-groomed appearance to sloppy attire, from orderly thinking to haphazard thought processes, from interest in everyday activities to an I-don't-care attitude. Food is left untouched, nights are spent sitting and staring out the window, while jobs go undone. There is lethargy, dejection, and often crying.

Once recognized, depression must be faced squarely. Start with a visit to the physician, who will begin counseling and perhaps prescribe an antidepressant drug such as amitriptyline (Elavil), imipramine (Tofranil), or doxepin (Sinequan or Adapin). Several days or weeks are needed to achieve the full benefit of medication, so be patient.

Depression often follows the relentless assault of daily duties—the ritual rising, the predictable problems, the constant chores, and the inevitable ennui at day's end. First-rate therapy often includes a change of scenery—a vacation trip to remove the individual from the tedium and stress of his life. In fact, hospitalization often represents just that, but a Caribbean trip is much more fun.

A new interest is an effective anidote against depression. How about oil painting (Churchill's choice), writing poetry, remodeling the bathroom, or planting a garden? Sometimes it helps to join a discussion or church group, as new friends open up hidden recesses of the personality.

Dealing with the depressed individual is hardly fun. His sense of gloom can depress all those about him and, in the end, only the most loyal of relatives and friends remain. But they will be rewarded, because almost without exception, the dark clouds lift and the once-depressed individual regains his zest for life again.

If you or someone in your family suffers depression and want to learn more, write to:

The American Mental Health Foundation
2 East 86th Street
New York, New York 10028

The National Association for Mental Health
1800 North Kent Street
Rosslyn Station
Arlington, Virginia 22209

The Suicide Threat

Depression carries the ever-present threat of suicide. The focus seems to turn from apathy to hopelessness and the depressed individual begins to think, "Life isn't worth living. Why should I go on?" Then it's time to call the doctor. The physician knows the danger, and will examine the patient promptly. Perhaps he will arrange for out-patient treatment, or hospitalization may be suggested. Whatever the proposed therapy, keep in close touch with the physician and follow his instructions to the letter—and don't hesitate to call him at any hour if self-destructive urges seem to have the upper hand.

DIABETES MELLITUS

Synonym: sugar diabetes

Almost one of every three Americans carries the gene of diabetes. Of course, not all of these individuals are or will become diabetic, yet there are presently 1.6 million diabetics in the United States and another two million individuals destined to develop diabetes.

Diabetes is a shortage of the hormone insulin, which sets off a chain reaction leading to severe metabolic upheaval. Insulin, produced in the pancreas gland and released into the bloodstream, transports sugar from the blood into body cells where it is needed for energy. With insulin in short supply, sugar accumulates in the bloodstream, sometimes attaining gargantuan levels, and is discharged into the urine. The cells, on the other hand, are sugar-poor; weakness results and the body burns fats and protein for fuel.

The undue breakdown of body protein and fat creates an excess of acid byproducts, which are released into the bloodstream. As acidity of the blood rises, breathing may become deep (as the body tries to expel acid wastes as carbon dioxide) and mental acuity may falter. Eventually, a diabetic coma may result.

Yet, most of the more than three million actual and potential diabetics will never experience this succession of events. Instead, diabetes will be detected upon routine examination in the doctor's office, with therapy instituted to forestall the metabolic crisis that may attend untreated diabetes mellitus.

Detecting Diabetes

Finding the disease is the first step in self-help care. Important symptoms of diabetes are excessive appetite (as body cells clamor for sugar for energy), frequent passages of large amounts of urine (as sugar-laden urine draws fluid from the blood), and excessive thirst (as the body calls for replacement of fluid lost via urination). Other complaints may include lethargy due to sugar-poor cells; itching of the skin, perhaps due to sugar deposition; and visual changes as the fluid content of the eye's lens fluctuates.

Initial testing includes a urine analysis that reveals the presence of sugar. This can be done at home using Tes-Tape, available without prescription at the pharmacy. The physician may perform a blood test, usually showing the diabetic's blood sugar to be in excess of 130 mg per 100 cc when the individual is fasting, or above 170 mg per 100 cc when the specimen is taken following a meal. The height of the blood sugar count helps determine the treatment prescribed.

Treatment

Therapy of diabetes includes diet, pills, and insulin, as well as regular checkups by the physician to guide treatment and provide month-by-month follow-up. More than half of all diabetics can be treated by diet alone, and approximately another one-fifth will require supplemental oral medication. But if diet and pill therapy fail, then the physician will often prescribe insulin injections.

Diet therapy in diabetes has two goals: to attain and hold the ideal weight and to lessen the sugar load that the body must metabolize. Overweight individuals are encouraged to reduce to a predetermined goal prescribed by the physician. Quick starvation diets are inadvisable, since they may boost the blood acidity. Much better is a gradual weight reduction to a trim silhouette.

Reducing the sugar load cuts the need for insulin. As weight falls and metabolic demands slacken, the use of antidiabetic pills can sometimes be discontinued. Often prescribed for the unstable diabetic is the exchange diet, a highly precise but somewhat complicated computation based upon prescribed values of fats, protein, carbohydrates, and calories. For detailed instructions, contact your physician, the hospital dietitian, or write to:

American Diabetes Association, Inc.
18 East 48th Street
New York, New York 10017

The mild diabetic or the prediabetic showing only an occasional blood sugar peak may not require superstrict dietary diligence. More realistic may be a low carbohdyrate diet such as the following.

Low Carbohydrate Diet

Foods Permitted	*Foods to Be Avoided*

Cereals

Cooked oat and wheat cereals	Sugar-coated cereals
Dry precooked cereals	
Bran cereals	

Breads

2 slices daily of white or whole wheat bread	Muffins, rolls, and biscuits
Corn bread	Pancakes and waffles

Soups

Meat stock soups	Creamed soups
Bean, lentil, or split pea soups	
Bouillon and broth	

Meat, Fish, and Dairy Products

Boiled, baked, or broiled veal, ham, lean beef, turkey, chicken, fish, mutton, and pork	Fried or fatty meats
Shellfish	Fried eggs
Softcooked eggs	
Cheese	
Cottage cheese	

Vegetables

Cucumbers	Brussels Sprouts
Carrots	Turnips
Onions	Potatoes
Lettuce	Corn
Peas	Squash
Spinach	
Radishes	
Tomatoes	
Cabbage	
Beets	
Celery	
Asparagus	
Green beans	

Foods Permitted	Foods to Be Avoided

Fruits

Fruit juices	Dates
Apples	Pineapple
Bananas	Melons
Apricots	
Pears	
Prunes	
Oranges	
Grapefruit	
Plums	
Peaches	
Figs	
Raisins	

Desserts

Gelatin	Cakes
Dietetic desserts	Pies and pastries
	Custard and pudding
	Ice cream
	Sherbet
	Bread pudding
	Tapioca pudding
	Corn starch or rice pudding

Beverages

Coffee, tea	Carbonated beverages
Decaffeinated coffee	Alcohol
Cocoa, Postum, and Ovaltine	
Milk	
Skimmed milk	
Buttermilk	

Miscellaneous

Liquid vegetable oils (corn, soybean, and safflower)	Animal fats and lard
Salt	Sugar
Pepper	Nuts
Olives	Macaroni and spaghetti
Pickles	Mayonnaise
Tomato paste	Gravy
Garlic	Jelly and jam
Mustard	Candy
Horseradish	Honey and molasses
Relish	
Vinegar	

Antidiabetic Medication

Antidiabetic pills lower blood sugar levels and help many mild diabetics avoid insulin therapy. Two general types are available:

- Sulfonylurea agents are offspring of sulfanilamide that spur the pancreas to produce insulin while slowing release of sugar from the liver. In this family are tolbutamide (Orinase), tolazamide (Tolinase), chlorpropamide (Diabinese), and acetohexamide (Dymelor).
- Diguanide antidiabetic therapy offers only one choice; phenformin (DBI. Available as tablets or as a time release capsule, phenformin enhances sugar metabolism in the tissues and lowers glucose output by the liver.

There is some difference of opinion among specialists as to the efficacy of these compounds. One group of physicians claim, "They're no better than diet alone." And recent studies suggest that there may be more cardiac deaths among patients who use antidiabetic oral medication. Opponents assert, "The study method was biased, and results are inconclusive." Until the dust settles, your own physician is the best source of advice concerning oral antidiabetic agents.

Insulin therapy is needed for the hard-to-manage adult-onset diabetic and for virtually all juvenile-onset diabetics (who classically suffer a more stormy course than their adult counterparts). Given in one or two injections each day, insulin is obtainable in both rapid-acting and longer-acting forms that can be administered independently or combined in the same syringe. Available are the following preparations:

- Regular insulin, also called crystalline insulin, acts within one hour and is out of the body within eight hours. It is used for rapid action, when minute-by-minute control is needed, and sometimes is mixed with longer-acting preparations to stabilize bounding blood sugar levels.
- NPH insulin and Lente insulin have similar properties and are the most widely used types of insulin. Following injection, a peak of activity is reached in 8 to 10

hours, although some insulin action persists for about 24 hours.

- Protamine-zinc insulin is seldom used, since it exerts its maximum effect at 12 to 18 hours, and may cause middle-of-the-night insulin reactions.

Insulin Reactions

The diabetic taking insulin must ever be wary of the insulin reaction. It begins insidiously and progresses much more rapidly than the development of diabetic coma, although relief may be attained within minutes if the correct diagnosis is made and therapy started immediately.

Here's the usual story: Diabetic Harry Atkinson overslept and ate only a light breakfast, but took his usual morning dose of 44 units of NPH insulin. For one reason or another he skipped lunch altogether, and at about 4 P.M. he suddenly felt weak, shaky, jittery, and sweaty. Fortunately, Harry recognized the symptoms and gulped a glass of orange juice laced with sugar to combat the effects of hypoglycemia (q.v.).

If untreated, however, hypoglycemia can progress to loss of consciousness, and injection therapy is then needed to boost blood sugar levels and prevent possible brain damage. The physician may inject glucose (sugar) intravenously, but this type of administration is technically difficult. Much easier and eminently safe is the injection of Glucagon, easily prepared by a household member following the package instructions and injected virtually anywhere into the body. Glucagon boosts blood sugar levels temporarily and the patient usually soon recovers consciousness, following which oral feedings are resumed. If you are a diabetic taking insulin, ask your physician if perhaps a vial of Glucagon should be kept with your insulin syringe.

What You Can Do about Diabetes

Unquestionably, the diabetic and his physician are partners in management of the disease. There will be regular checkups, blood tests, diet advice, and perhaps prescriptions for pills or insulin. But there's much the patient can do to learn about diabetes and to forestall its complications.

- Stay slim. Some folks seem to eat themselves into diabetes, and weight control might have delayed the onset of the disease for decades.
- Go for regular checkups, particularly if there is a family history of diabetes. The symptoms we have mentioned may be present if the blood sugar level is high, but mild cases often display no symptoms and it is better to detect diabetes on routine physical examination than lapse into diabetic coma during a viral flu.
- Don't deviate from the doctor's dietary advice. He has calculated the correct diet for your age, weight, activity, and blood sugar level. You have paid for his advice; now follow it.
- If you take insulin or antidiabetic pills, carry a card, bracelet, or locket identifying you as a diabetic. A good source is Medic Alert, P. O. Box 1009, Turlock, California, 95380. Approved by more than 100 organizations, including the prestigious American Academy of Family Physicians, the Medic Alert Foundation provides an emergency file on each member, listing diseases such as diabetes, allergies, the patient's nearest relative, and private physician. Members receive a medallion or bracelet and a wallet-size identification card telling the chief medical problem plus the member's identification number and the round-the-clock Medic Alert emergency telephone number.
- Diabetics should learn to test their urine each day, using a Tes-Tape quick dip-stick test for urinary glucose or other test method that the doctor may recommend.
- Learn proper care of the feet, since diabetics suffer increased hardening of the arteries to the legs. Foot infections may prove difficult to cure, yet could have been avoided by proper foot care.
- Learn all you can about diabetes. Read books, starting with this one, magazine articles, pamphlets in the doctor's office, and anything you see in print about diabetes. The older diabetic should read Chapter 19 of *Feeling Alive after 65* (Arlington House .Publishers, New Rochelle, New York).
- Learn more; a pioneering center in diabetes research

and treatment is The Joslin Diabetes Foundation, 15 Joslin Road, Boston, Massachusetts 02215. Patients returning from a few days here have a heightened understanding of their disease.

The diabetic learns to live with his disease. He must. But with attention to diet and weight control, the frequent medical checkups demanded by the disease, and the ever-increasing arsenal of weapons against it, many diabetics will outlive their nondiabetic peers!

DIAPER RASH

Synonym: diaper dermatitis

It's really no wonder that most babies suffer, now and again, from diaper dermatitis. Soap dissolved in cloth diapers, urine and feces held against the infant's bottom, the inevitable plastic pants that block out fresh air—all these combine to irritate the baby's naturally tender skin.

Diaper rash begins as a faint red irritation as urine and alkaline soap particles dissolve the protective skin oils. Once the skin's protective mantle is gone, irritants go to work on skin cells beneath, producing redness, swelling, and intense discomfort. Before long bacteria, ringworm fungi, or yeastlike Candida discover the irritated area and set up housekeeping there.

What to Do about Diaper Rash

In medical school, young physicians are taught, "First of all, do no harm to your patient." Mothers, be sure that *you* are not causing the diaper rash. A common cause of diaper dermatitis is soap caked on improperly washed diapers. The proud young mother wants her infant attired in the whitest diapers in town, and she loads her washer with extra-strong detergent. The first gush of urine dissolves residual soap particles from the diaper, and these go to work on baby's skin. If you do your own diapers, use no soap other than Ivory Snow or Fels Naptha. Use a little less than you think you should; then be sure to run the diapers through a second rinse in the washing machine. Bleaches make the diapers white, but can intensify diaper dermatitis; fabric softeners don't help matters either.

How about paper diapers? These, too, will produce diaper rashes from time to time, if wet or soiled diapers are not changed promptly. Although diaper services always had a good record in preventing diaper rash, paper diapers seem to be driving diaper services from the American scene.

Change the diaper promptly when soiled or wet, lest baby's skin suffer the irritant effect of urine or feces. It may mean getting out of bed at night, but that beats treating a diaper dermatitis.

Mild diaper rashes usually respond to over-the-counter medication. A time-honored favorite is Desitin ointment containing zinc oxide, lanolin, cod liver oil, petrolatum, and talcum. Another first-rate product is Johnson's Baby Cream, which contains mineral oil, lanolin, paraffin, and white bee's wax ceresin. My favorite has been Acid Mantle Cream containing aluminum acetate, and for resistant diaper irritation I often prescribe ⅛-percent Cort-Dome Cream containing ⅛-percent micronized hydrocortisone alcohol in Acid Mantle Cream.

Baby powders won't cure diaper rash, but they may help absorb the moisture of urine and perspiration. Two good ones are Mennen Baby Magic Powder containing methylbenzethonium chloride plus talc, and Johnson's Medicated Powder containing talc and calcium silicate.

A topical antibiotic preparation such as Bacitracin Ointment is available without prescription and will eradicate tiny islands of bacterial infection that may complicate a diaper rash. Following each diaper change, apply the Bacitracin Ointment only to areas of infection—it's not intended for use on ordinary diaper dermatitis.

Prescription medication is needed when self-help remedies fail. Perhaps a lingering infection is caused by a Candida (monilia) infection with a magenta-colored sheen to the skin, surrounded by tiny satellite islands of infection. For this, the doctor will probably prescribe a nystatin (Mycostatin) cream. Or perhaps there is a ringworm fungus infection that may respond to nonprescription therapy with tolnaftate (Tinactin) cream. Or a stubborn bacterial infection may respond only to oral antibiotics and a potent antibiotic cream such as gentamycin (Garamycin) cream or ointment.

EAR INFECTIONS

Synonyms: otitis externa, otitis media

Ear infections are common disorders of children, but can occur at any age. Two distinct types are found, although they may coexist in the same individual: Otitis media is an infection of the middle ear, and otitis externa involves the ear canal plus perhaps the outer ear.

Otitis Externa

External ear infections often follow swimming or the injudicious insertion of cotton-tipped applicators or hairpins into the ear canal. The symptoms are itching and pain in the ear canal, perhaps associated with a puslike discharge.

Where external ear infections are concerned, self-help concerns prevention. Those prone to ear canal infections should wear a tight bathing cap while swimming and perhaps also use ear plugs. Deep diving under the water must be avoided, since this drives water into the ear canal under pressure. And, of course, as the old adage runs, the ear canal should be invaded by nothing smaller than the elbow.

If symptoms of an ear canal disorder are noted, see the dcotor promptly. There is no home remedy or over-the-counter prescription that will arrest the infection.

Otitis Media

The middle ear infection usually follows a cold, during which bacteria from the throat enter the middle ear via the Eustachian tube. Once inside the middle ear cavity, germs multiply, causing severe pain perhaps associated with impaired hearing. Fever is often present, and there will be drainage from the ear if the eardrum is perforated by rising pressure.

Middle ear infections can sometimes be prevented. Never swim (and most especially never dive deep below the surface) if a common cold is present. Also the patient with a common cold should not ride in an airplane, since changing air pressures promote the migration of bacteria from the throat to the middle ear. Cold victims should treat their illnesses: the use of a decongestant such as a pseudoephedrine (Sudafed) 30-mg tablet taken four times daily, and ¼-percent phenylephrine (Neo-Synephrine) nosedrops in each nostril three times daily helps clear passageways and may prevent a middle ear infection.

But if infection occurs, see the physician. He will prescribe an antibiotic such as penicillin for the infection, probably accompanied by a decongestant to open the Eustachian tubes, and will probably recommend follow-up visits until any lost hearing acuity has been regained.

ECZEMA

Synonym: atopic dermatitis

In 543 A.D. the word eczema was coined from a Greek term *ekzein* meaning to boil out, and since then the catchall diagnosis of eczema has been applied to almost every chronic skin disease known to man.

Usually involving the flexor surface of the body—the crease behind the ears, the front of the elbows and wrists, and behind the knees—eczema causes a red, intensely itching rash. Scratching begets more itching, and the end result may be a chronic thickened intractably irritating dermatitis.

Three factors appear to play a role in eczema. Almost all individuals who contact it come from families with a history of allergies. Perhaps a sibling suffered skin rashes in infancy, an aunt had childhood asthma, and a cousin is taking shots for bee-sting allergy. Secondly, flare-ups of eczema may follow overindulgence in highly allergenic foods such as chocolate, nuts, berries, or tomato products. Finally, there are emotions, the sparks of nervous energy that can set an eczematous rash ablaze.

Eliminating Eczema

The genetic heritage of the eczema victim can't be changed, but he can curtail his contact with problem-causing sources of allergy. Eczema may follow eating a chocolate bar, washing with a perfumed soap, or taking a dose of penicillin. Or perhaps the cause is obscure, such as an allergy to ubiquitous ingredients such as milk, eggs, or wheat (see the food allergy elimination list on page 120). Skin testing by the physician may be needed to pinpoint causes of allergy-induced eczema flare-ups.

Emotions must be controlled. Anxiety-producing situations should be avoided, responsibility reduced, and some relief may follow use of one of the nonprescription antihistamine sedatives such as Cope or Compoz.

Local therapy of eczema may include over-the-counter preparations such as Acid Mantle Cream, containing aluminum acetate, or a tar-based preparation such as Tar-Doak Lotion, containing 5 percent tar distillate. Nevertheless, the most effective antieczema preparations are such prescription-only cortisone compounds as betamethasone valerate (Valisone) cream or ointment; fluocinolone (Synalar) cream, ointment, or solution; or fluocinonide (Lidex) cream or ointment.

Cortisone by pills or by injection may be prescribed for severe eczema. Usually recommended as short-term therapy, cortisone can dramatically clear eczema in widespread areas, although the dermatitis may return when cortisone administration ceases.

EMPHYSEMA

Synonym: pulmonary emphysema

Emphysema is on the rise. This chronic, debilitating lung disease is becoming more prevalent each day as air pollution takes its toll and more and more packs of cigarettes are consumed each year. The disease attacks the entire respiratory system (see Figure 10), with most damage occurring in the lung's tiny alveolar air sacs.

Emphysema does not emerge suddenly, but develops gradually over years and even decades, as chronic allergic congestion, respiratory irritation due to pollutants, and chronic bronchitis cause repeated bouts of coughing. In time, colds lead to lung infections, with fever, chest congestion, and an occasional full-blown pneumonia. With each chest cold and pneumonia, and indeed with each cough, a few tiny air sacs (alveoli) in the lungs are damaged.

The alveoli—the business part of the lung—are millions of

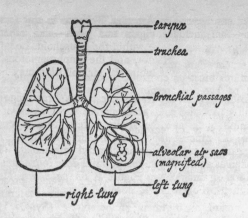

FIGURE 10. *The respiratory system.*

tiny air sacs separated by tissue paper-thin walls. In the alveoli, oxygen passes into the blood coursing through tiny vessels in the walls, and the same blood gives up carbon dioxide wastes that are expelled with the next breath. As emphysema advances, each cough breaks the walls of a few tiny efficient alveoli, and left behind is a larger, less efficient, flabby sac. Eventually, there are few remaining walls between the large alveolar sacs; little oxygen is picked up, and carbon dioxide wastes accumulate. Complicating this failure of pulmonary function is a chronic hacking cough, often bringing up thick mucus.

The emphysema patient complains of shortness of breath. He is often "winded" after only slight exertion and may struggle to breathe when quiet. You will see him sitting with elbows braced on the table, so that he can use a few extra shoulder and chest muscles to augment breathing.

Treatment

Therapy of emphysema includes attempts to slow progress of the disease, removal of phlegm, opening of airways, control of infection, medication prescribed by the physician, and breathing exercises.

Bronchial irritants must be removed from the atmosphere. Most important is tobacco smoke, the prime cause of most cases of emphysema in America. Tobacco in any form is forbidden—that includes cigars and pipes—and other family members must not smoke within the household. Local air pollution may also be a factor, and the emphysematous individual living in an area of industrial air pollution may be forced to move.

Clearing phlegm from the chest aids breathing. Chronic bronchitis precedes and accompanies most cases of pulmonary emphysema, and the victim suffers from excessive production of mucus that can impair breathing. A good expectorant to cut phlegm is glyceryl guaiacolate (Robitussin) taken as a one- to two-teaspoonful dose four times daily.

Postural drainage (see Figure 8 on page 56) also helps clear mucus. Following a dose of glyceryl guaiacolate, lie over the edge of the bed with the elbows on the floor and head dependent. Give several good coughs, then turn to the right, next to the left. Gravity helps drain phlegm from hidden recesses of the lungs and can aid breathing throughout the remainder of the day.

Sometimes there is bronchial spasm, and difficult breathing may be episodic, just as the asthmatic suffers acute shortness of breath from time to time. In these cases asthma remedies may be helpful, including Bronkolixer, containing ephedrine sulfate, glyceryl guaiacolate, theophylline, and phenobarbital, in a dose of two teaspoonfuls three or four times daily. Also available are Tedral Tablets containing ephedrine hydrochloride, theophylline, and phenobarbital; one tablet may be taken every four to six hours for shortness of breath associated with wheezing. Before using these medicines, it's best to check with your physician.

Antibiotics are prescribed when infection is present. Tetracycline is a favorite, and sometimes the doctor will recommend long-term use, with the drug taken four times daily, Monday, Tuesday, and Wednesday, and the next four days a treatment-free period.

Inhalation therapy is sometimes prescribed, and there is no place for self-help oxygen use here, since the indiscriminate administration of oxygen can cause breathing problems in advanced emphysema. In addition to prescribing the type of inhalation therapy, the doctor will often write a prescription for medication to be added to the inhaler, helping to dissolve phlegm and to open bronchial passageways during inhalation therapy.

Inhalers are used when bronchial spasm blocks the flow of air. Available without prescription is Bronkaid Aerosol Mist containing epinephrine. Or the physician may prescribe Duo-Medihaler, an aerosol device that effectively opens congested bronchial passages.

Breathing exercises can be done at home to open idle alveoli and release trapped air, and to strengthen the diaphragm and associated muscles of respiration (see Figure 11). Begin gradually, increasing repetitions slowly until each exercise is repeated 20 times morning and night:

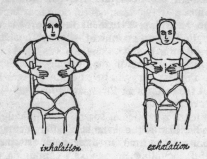

inhalation   *exhalation*

Chest compression to expel stale air.

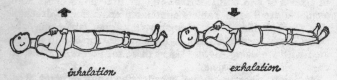

inhalation   *exhalation*

Strengthening the diaphragm.

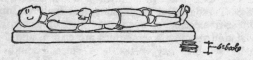

Building the respiratory muscles.

FIGURE 11. *Breathing exercises.*

- Exercise 1 removes stale air. Sit straight in a firm chair, and place your hands over the lower ribs. Breathe deeply, feeling your lungs expand. Then exhale completely, compressing the chest wall with your hands.
- Exercise 2 builds the muscles of the diaphragm. Lie flat on your back with left hand on your chest and right hand on the abdomen. Inhale deeply, trying to raise the hand on the abdomen without expanding the chest—i.e., breathe with the abdomen, inhaling rapidly through the nose and exhaling slowly through pursed lips.
- Exercise 3 further strengthens the chest muscles and diaphragm. Lie supine on bed with the foot of the bed raised six inches on books or a chair. Instead of a hand, place a weight on the abdomen; a filled rubber water bottle or encyclopedia volume is about heavy enough. Inhale, raising the weight, then exhale slowly as the weight falls.

A first-rate illustrated booklet is *Living with Asthma, Chronic Bronchitis, and Emphysema*, available from:

Riker Laboratories
Northridge, California 91324

EYE INJURIES

Synonyms: particle in the eye, foreign substances in the eye, scratched eye

The eye—our window to the world—is as delicate and fragile as crystal, and a small injury can cause a major disability. There are three minor eye problems that can often be managed at home.

Particle in the Eye

A speck of dust, wood, or metal may lodge in the eye; it feels like a huge boulder, and its significance depends upon its location and the ease of removal.

Specks under the lower lid are almost always easily removed with a moist cotton-tipped applicator (Q-tip or its equivalent).

More difficult to dislodge are particles under the upper lid. Mother's trick of lifting the upper lid and pulling it down over the lower lid is sometimes successful, as the lower lashes sweep away the speck under the upper lid. If this fails, it will be necessary to turn the upper lid inside out, using the wooden end of a cotton-tipped applicator to press down about ⅜ inch from the edge while the lid margin and lashes are folded up. It's a technically easy procedure *if* you have been shown how, and it usually reveals the speck under the upper lid.

Particles under both lower and upper lids are often washed away when the eye is flushed with ordinary tap water or with nonprescription Dacriose Solution of boric acid, potassium chloride, and sodium carbonate in a jet-stream spray bottle.

The foreign body imbedded in the cornea (clear area over the iris of the eye) is often quite painful and hard to dislodge. Especially troublesome is the speck of iron that can form a rust ring. A gentle attempt may be made to dislodge the particle with Dacriose Solution or a moistened cotton-tipped applicator; however, if not immediately successful, desist and call the doctor.

Foreign Substance in the Eye

As flowers attract bees, the eye seems to attract soapy water, gasoline, cleansers, and other fluids. Local irritation is common and is usually the only result. Most dangerous are strong alkali or acid solutions, which could cause permanent damage to the cornea.

When a foreign substance splashes into the eye, it should be washed away as soon as possible. Good first aid is Dacriose Jet-Stream Spray, but also effective is flushing with tap water: turn your head upside down under the tap. Continue gently washing for five minutes, followed by a call to the doctor if the offending solution was alkali, acid, or other potentially damaging chemical.

Scratched Eye

Common causes of a scratched eye include tree branches, thrown objects, and fingernails (often of an infant). If the eye is merely bruised, even with a "blood spot" of the white area, no active treatment is needed.

A scratch of the cornea, however, is more troublesome—painful and a potential source of visual impairment if infection and scarring occur. The doctor treats a corneal abrasion by patching to keep the eye closed, and healing is usually complete within a day or two. The presence of infection in a corneal abrasion, signaled by excruciating pain and sensitivity to light, requires aggressive therapy including antibiotics.

FAINTING

Synonym: syncope

Fainting is a sudden loss of consciousness, and may accompany any combination of prolonged standing, low blood sugar (such as missing a meal), anxiety, fever, flu, stuffy atmosphere, fright, anemia, a hot humid day, or any of a dozen other causes. The episode usually occurs with little warning. Color drains from the face, the individual becomes suddenly quiet, then slumps to the floor.

Little need be done in the self-help treatment of syncope. By dropping to the floor, the individual has assumed the optimum position, allowing maximum blood flow to the brain. First aid includes only protecting the victim from harm, perhaps loosening a tight collar, maintaining body warmth, and possibly elevating the feet to assure blood flow to vital organs. The skin will feel moist and cool to the touch, returning to its normal dry warmth as consciousness returns.

A finger on the pulse is reassurance that a regular heart beat exists, and assures more ambitious onlookers that "something is being done." Above all, the self-helper must restrain the energetic individual who feels compelled to pour hot coffee or whiskey down the victim's throat or stand him on his feet.

Almost without exception, the fainting individual will recover consciousness within a few minutes. Encourage him to remain horizontal for a short time more, lest lightheadedness accompany his efforts to stand. When the pulse is slow, the skin warm and dry, and alertness complete, the patient may be allowed to sit in a chair and sip a high-calorie drink, such as fruit juice laced with sugar.

115

If the cause of fainting is known, such as sitting in a stuffy room after skipping breakfast or fainting following a sudden fright, then nothing else need be done; however, if the cause of syncope is obscure, a visit to the doctor may be in order.

FEVER

Synonym: pyrexia

Fever is an elevation of the body's temperature above 100°F (37.6°C). The presence of a fever suggests that some disorder is present, whether infection, dehydration, blood disease, malignancy, or any of a host of other maladies. Fever, in itself, is not a diagnosis, but a symptom of disease.

The body temperature fluctuates from hour to hour during the day, often lowest in the morning, peaking in the late afternoon, then dropping during the evening hours. Not uncommonly, individuals record this daily variation and conclude that they have an afternoon "fever," although the temperature never exceeds 100°F.

A fever of moderate height (up to 102°F) and of short duration (less than 24 hours) in an individual who otherwise appears well is probably due to a mild infection, will probably be self-limited, and is initially best managed by aspirin and observation. A rising temperature, the onset of other symptoms such as vomiting or cough, or persistence of the fever suggest that the doctor should be called.

FINGERTIP INJURIES

Synonyms: crushed finger, fingernail injury, subungual hematoma

Fingertip injuries occur in car doors, dresser drawers, and under heavy objects. The tissues suffer bruising (see Bruise), the bone may be damaged, and a blood clot often forms beneath the nail.

Self-help therapy begins with application of ice packs during the first 24 hours, followed by warm soaks after the first day. Cold helps reduce initial swelling, and later warm soaks

(30 to 60 minutes four times daily) increase blood flow to aid healing.

Injured bones should be splinted. A Popsicle stick works well for older children and adults; a paperclip is a useful splint for a toddler's finger. Severe pain suggests a possible fracture; see the doctor for an x-ray.

A blood clot under the nail (subungual hematoma) should be evacuated—to relieve pain and hopefully to prevent loss of the fingernail. The technique I employ in my office can be used at home; all you need is a paperclip and cigarette lighter. Scrub the nail, allow the area to dry, then hold the finger firmly on the table. Unfold the paperclip so that one end is extended, then heat this end with the cigarette lighter until it is red hot. Next, gently press the hot paperclip end through the nail into the center of the clot. Pain is minimal; the nail is insensitive, and the blood clot dissipates the heat so that the nail bed feels little discomfort. (Really!) I have a $15 nail drill that I no longer use, since the hot paperclip method is much faster and less painful.

After draining a subungual hematoma, it's important to soak the fingertip in warm salt water for 30 minutes four times daily.

FISHHOOK INJURIES

Although Mom is the first-aider treating most minor injuries, removal of an imbedded fishhook is often Dad's duty. He and Junior are off to spend the day together fishing. Bait the hook, give one good cast, and—POW!—the fishhook is imbedded in the scalp, finger, forearm, or what-have-you.

There are several ways to handle fishhook injuries. Method one is to advance the hook so that the point emerges from the skin, leaving a wound of entry and exit. Then grasp the point and barb with pliers, clip below the barb with wire cutters, and pull the hook back through. The advantage of this method is a minimum of tissue tearing with the barb. The disadvantages? There's a second puncture of the skin, and the wire cutters that will snip the fishhook are probably back home in the workshop.

My favorite method is quick removal of the hook, barb and all, back through the wound of entry. In my family practice office, I scrub and sterilize with povidone-iodine (Betadine), then inject a local anesthetic, clamp the hook securely, and pull quickly! The barb makes the pull a little more difficult, but causes negligible tissue injury.

Of course, when fishing, there's no anesthetic available, and the best antiseptic may be soap and water or perhaps a little whiskey you had along "for medicinal purposes." Then try the New England fisherman'a adaptation of my simple fishhook removal method: Tie a loop of string or fishing line about 20 inches in diameter. Place the loop around the hook and the right hand within the loop; steady the base of the hook with the left hand. Then quickly and firmly snap the heel of the hand against the end of the loop as shown in Figure 12, deftly removing the fishhook from the skin. Following removal of the fishhook, the area should be scrubbed thoroughly, and this is repeated upon arrival home, followed by a warm salt-water soak (one teaspoonful of table salt in a pint of warm water) for 30 minutes four times daily. And check with the physician to see if Junior's tetanus booster is up to date.

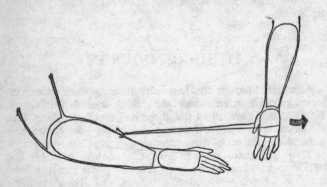

FIGURE 12. *How New England fishermen remove a fishhook.*

FLATFOOT

Synonym: pes planus
The flatfoot deformity is really the heel and forefoot roll-

ing under and out, obliterating the arch and sometimes causing discomfort by abnormal weight distribution at the ankle. Pes planus is often hereditary, and the individual whose arch is flat as a pancake probably has one or more relatives with the same affliction.

Treatment

There's no cure for the flatfoot deformity, but intrinsic muscles of the foot can be strengthened by the following exercise: Place a pencil on the floor, then try to pick up the pencil by curling the toes. Perform this maneuver for 10 repetitions four times daily.

Foot and ankle discomfort is avoided by normalizing the stress placed upon these areas. Arch supports—called scaphoid pads—are incorporated into each new pair of shoes, and sometimes recommended is a Thomas heel to support the inner heel bone of the flat foot.

FOOD ALLERGIES

Food allergies can occur at any age, from infancy to the senior years. Crying and cramps characterize the milk intolerance of infants; preschool children may complain of abdominal discomfort, perhaps associated with vomiting or diarrhea. In older and more articulate individuals, symptoms of food allergy may be described as abdominal distress, loose bowel movements, periodic vomiting, headache, muscular pains, or aching joints. In some individuals skin manifestations occur, notably hives or eczema.

What to Do about Food Allergies

The best diagnostic tool, and one often advised by the physician, is the diet diary. A twenty-five-cent notebook is all that's needed: Each time symptoms occur, jot down the time of day, and all foods eaten during the preceding six to eight hours. Include everything; don't edit out favorite treats. Before long a pattern will emerge. Perhaps abdominal distress comes after eating catsup or tomato paste. Maybe the culprit is peanuts, found in more than one hundred common house-

Begin by eliminating all foods in one or more of the following lists:

Food Allergy Elimination Diets

Wheat	Milk	Chocolate
Beer	Baked foods	Chocolate cake
Biscuits	Biscuits	Chocolate candy
Bread	Bologna	Chocolate and
Bread crumbs	Butter	chocolate chip
Candy	Candy	cookies
Cereals	Cheese	Chocolate custard
Chowders	Chocolate	Chocolate frosting
Crackers	Cocoa	Chocolate ice
Flour	Cream	cream
Frankfurters	Creamed soups	Chocolate milk
Gravy	Frankfurters	Cocoa
Macaroni	Gravy	
Noodles	Ice Cream	
Spaghetti	Margarine	
	Milk sherbets	
	Pudding	
	Scalloped foods	
	Waffles	
	White sauces	

Eggs	Tomatoes	Peanuts
Baked foods	Barbecue sauce	Crackerjack
Breads (check	Catsup	Earth nut
label)	Chicken cacciatore	Goober nut
Candy	Chili	Groundnut
Croquettes	Cocktail sauce	Margarine with
Custards	Lasagne	peanut oil
French ice cream	Moussaka	Monkey nut
French toast	Pizza	Peanut brittle
Fritters	Ravioli	Peanut butter
Frostings	Shrimp creole	Peanut candy
Hollandaise sauce	Spaghetti sauce	Peanut oil
Mayonnaise	Spanish rice	Roasted peanuts
Meringue	Stewed tomatoes	Salted peanuts
Noodles	Tomato juice	
Pancakes	Tomato paste	
Salad dressing	Tomato sauce	
Waffles	Veal parmesan	

hold foods. When and if the diet diary suggests the cause of food allergy, a trial at dietary elimination is warranted.

The following lists help pinpoint allergies and eliminate troublesome foods from the diet. For three weeks, omit all foods in one or more of the suspect lists; then reintroduce one list of foods, partaking generously of these foods for the next two weeks. If no symptoms occur during the two-week reintroduction period, the foods on that list are not the cause of the symptoms and a second list should be added for the next two weeks, and so forth. If the resumption of foods from the wheat, milk, or other list causes symptoms, then all foods in that group should be eliminated for at least six months. At the end of six months, the individual foods on the list may be added one at a time. Sometimes the allergy abates after the cause has been absent from the diet for six months.

Other possible causes of food allergy include berries (particularly strawberries), fruits (don't forget fruit punches), corn products, seafood (clams, oysters, etc.), or chicken. And don't overlook the possibility of medicine—including over-the-counter preparations—as a possible source of allergy.

Avoiding the offending allergen should be sufficient to prevent symptoms. Of course, when vital nutrients are eliminated from the diet, their absence must be replaced with vitamins and perhaps protein from other sources.

The physician should be consulted before embarking upon long-term dietary restrictions. He may also prescribe anticholinergic or antihistamine medication to minimize symptoms, and occasionally he will recommend desensitization injections, particularly when food sensitivity is but part of a serious allergy problem.

FOOD POISONING

Synonym: toxic gastroenteritis

Explosive vomiting, cramps, and diarrhea characterize food poisoning, and the most feared complication is dehydration, although most individuals recover spontaneously as soon as the ingested toxin is metabolized. Since few of us eat alone, true food poisoning usually afflicts several individuals who share a common bond of having eaten the tainted food.

Types of Food Poisoning

Food poisoning is a catchall term describing a number of various maladies:

- Botulism occurrs after eating the toxin of Clostridium botulinus in improperly canned foods. Botulinus poisoning is discussed in more detail on page 54.
- Staphylococcal food poisoning follows a classic pattern. A creamy confection, a tasty pudding, or a salad mixed with mayonnaise is prepared, then stored without refrigeration, allowing staph germs time to multiply and produce a toxin. Hours later the contaminated food is served to the family or perhaps at a church picnic on a Sunday afternoon. Within a few hours most individuals who sampled the food will suffer explosive vomiting, cramps, and diarrhea lasting a day or two.
- Insecticide on fruits picked right off the tree can cause abdominal cramps and vomiting. This poisoning is easily avoided by washing all fruit before eating.
- Mushroom poisoning causes typical gastrointestinal symptoms associated with salivation, profuse sweating, excitability, widely dilated pupils, and shortness of breath with wheezing. Once the cause is ascertained, the doctor will prescribe fluids plus atropine to combat the specific poisoning found in inedible mushrooms. Avoid mushroom poisoning by eating only commercially available mushrooms.
- Foreign substances may cause food poisoning with obscure symptoms and elusive origins. Cattle grazing on jimson weed or snake root may produce milk containing toxic substances. Silverware cleaned with cyanide may contain traces of this poison, and nitrate-producing soil bacteria may contaminate a poorly capped well.

What to Do about Food Poisoning

Many cases of food poisoning are mild; almost all will be self-limited, and self-help treatment will usually suffice. Take lukewarm fluids in small quantities—weak tea, Jello water, ginger ale, and thin bouillon. Avoid excessively hot or cold liquids, shun salt and seasoning, and defer solid food until the symptoms subside. When nausea and vomiting cease, add to the diet soft bland foods such as thick soup, chicken breast, hard-boiled eggs, mashed potato, and boiled rice.

Vomiting may be controlled with Emetrol (a solution of levulose and dextrose) taken in an adult dose of one or two tablespoonfuls every three to four hours if needed. No prescription is needed for Emetrol, nor for Donnagel, a combination of kaolin and belladonna derivatives. Donnagel controls cramps and diarrhea when taken in an adult dose of one or two tablespoonfuls three or four times daily.

Within 48 hours after their onset, the manifestations of food poisoning should be gone. If symptoms persist, or grow worse despite home treatment, intravenous fluids may be needed and the doctor should be called.

FRACTURE

Synonym: broken bone

Automobile accidents, household mishaps, and sports injuries are the chief causes of fractures. A forceful blow is needed to break a bone, and following the acute injury there is severe pain perhaps associated with deformity. Movement of a broken bone (which should be avoided) causes a grating sensation called crepitus. The patient is extremely reluctant to move the injured part, and ill-advised attempts to "reduce the fracture" or transport the patient without proper splinting can complicate an otherwise simple break.

Treatment

Self-help therapy of suspected fractures involves preventing further injury and securing medical attention. When dealing with a fracture, there is no substitute for judgement, and when a serious injury has occurred (as in an automobile accident), it is often best to make the patient comfortable where he lies and await arrival of skilled medical assistance. Injured skiers should not be moved until arrival of the ski patrol—trained to handle fractures with special splints that adapt to injured extremities. But sometimes it's necessary to take independent action, and in these cases the careful application of a home splint can facilitate transportation to the doctor's office or hospital.

A rolled magazine (see Figure 13) makes one of the best splints I know. The magazine is adapted to the injured part and taped or tied in place, perhaps secured with an Ace Bandage and/or supported with a sling.

Another good splint is an ordinary bed pillow, which can cushion and immobilize an injured foot or ankle. Gently snuggle the injured part in the pillow, then secure with adhesive tape.

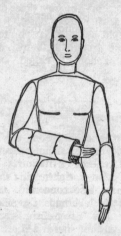

FIGURE 13. *Magazine splint.*

Ill-advised attempts at home reduction of fractures can cause permanent damage. Only an x-ray can detect the presence and extent of a broken bone, and definitive treatment should be undertaken only by a physician.

FRIGIDITY

Synonym: sexual dysfunction in the female

Failure of the female to achieve orgasm during sexual relations is defined as frigidity. Most women fail to reach a sex-

124

ual climax from time to time, many often, and some never reach climax. We are concerned here with the last two groups.

Rarely is the cause physical, although a vaginal irritation or tight vaginal tissues may be contributing factors. Far more common is failure of the couple to communicate in bed. In many cases, the husband has sex with his wife rather than making love with her. More quickly aroused than she, he proceeds pell-mell and ejaculates long before her interest is aroused. Not knowing or perhaps not caring about her responses, he may fail to provide the words of love and reassuring caresses that she craves.

Sometimes guilt feelings are her problem, perhaps springing from childhood suppositions that sex was evil. Perhaps guilt feelings spring from remorse about an indiscretion. In other women frigidity goes hand in hand with hostility, this woman denying her husband the satisfaction of responding to his ardent efforts.

Overcoming Frigidity

When frigidity cools the bedroom, see the doctor. He will perform a thorough physical examination, and prescribe treatment for any vaginal irritation while recommending methods to relieve undue tightness. Discuss your problem frankly, and ask his advice concerning sexual techniques to overcome erotic inertia. Perhaps the physician will suggest that the husband be present at the next interview, since frigidity is a problem for both man and wife.

When the husband understands his wife's slower sexual responses, her need for words of endearment and knowledge that he cares about her as a person, sex is often better than before, and more likely to be climaxed by orgasm.

A few technical tips may help. Sometimes a drink before love-making is relaxing, or perhaps an evening together at the movies. A motel weekend can turn on a wife who feels trapped by diapers and dishes at home. During sex it helps if the husband will slow down, spending more time in foreplay to awaken his wife's sexual responses. It helps if she tells him what she finds exciting, and a few shared words can go a long way toward overcoming frigidity.

Frigidity should not be accepted, and answers should be

sought. Masters and Johnson have been quoted as saying, "Couples who can communicate in the bedroom can usually communicate outside of it." And a mutually satisfactory sexual relationship plays a vital role in a successful marriage.

Further information concerning sexuality and sex counseling is available from:

American Association of Sex Educators, Counselors, and Therapists
Suite 304
5010 Wisconsin Ave., N.W.
Washington, D.C. 20016

Sex Information and Education Council of the U.S.
137 North Franklin Street
Hempstead, New York 11550

FROSTBITE

Frostbite, like a burn, is an injury following exposure to extremes of temperature, and may result in loss of tissue. The severity of frostbite is determined by the outdoor temperature, cooling winds, presence of moisture, protection afforded by clothing, and the duration of exposure. When frostbite occurs, the skin is numb and yellow-white. Most commonly involved are toes, fingers, and the nose. At a ski resort, one day last winter, the ski patrol checked cheeks and noses of everyone leaving the chairlift and sent several unsuspecting early frostbite victims to the warming hut. All who live in areas where winter brings Jack Frost's nip should know how to prevent and treat frostbite.

Preventing Frostbite

During cold winter weather it pays to plan ahead. Loose, warm, windproof clothing helps prevent thermal damage to the skin and underlying tissues. Down, furs, foam, and wool best preserve body warmth, and dryness is assured by a waterproof outer layer. Damp clothing should be changed promptly, since moisture speeds heat loss.

Gloves, like clothing, should have an insulating inner core

covered by waterproof material. At subzero temperatures, metal should never be handled without gloves.

Petroleum byproducts are first-class insulators, and a light layer of Vaseline petroleum jelly or ordinary mineral oil may protect exposed facial tissues from windburn and frostbite. A more elegant preparation is Bonne Bell Weatherproofer, a favorite of skiers whose skin suffers all-day exposure to cold and wind.

Exercise increases circulation to hands and feet. When frostbite threatens, keep active, wiggle the fingers and toes, jump up and down, and (an old skier's method) rotate the arms at shoulders to speed blood to icy fingertips.

Treating Frostbite

Frostbite causes tissue injury that can be minimized by prompt *informed* action—or aggravated by overenthusiastic home treatment attempts. Frostbitten areas should be thawed and warmed promptly, yet carefully, lest overheating burn damaged areas; frostbitten tissues may suffer thermal burns at heating temperatures that would be safe for normal skin.

Warm hands and feet in a cozy warm blanket, in warm (but not hot) water, or, if no external source of heat is available, cover the nose with a warm hand or tuck frosty fingertips into the underarms. Don't rub or slap "to stimulate circulation," since this may cause tissue damage.

Sometimes frostbite occurs in remote areas, and if help is many miles away, it may be best to allow extremities to remain frozen. This helps assure circulation to the heart and vital organs, and may prevent damage to frozen extremities, since walking on a thawed foot may be more traumatic than bearing weight on a frozen one.

Once self-help first aid is begun, arrange emergency transportation to the nearest hospital, where the physician can begin his phase of the therapy of frostbite.

FUNGUS INFECTIONS

Synonyms: ringworm, athlete's foot, dermatophytosis

Ringworm fungus infections are as common as crabgrass, afflicting millions of Americans each year. Found in moist areas of the body and most prevalent during the hot summer months, fungus most often infects the feet, scalp, and warm, inviting skin folds.

Ringworm of the Feet

Ringworm of the feet, known to all as athlete's foot, is a fungus infection usually occurring between the toes and spreading to the tougher skin of the top and sole of the foot. The infection is often acquired by walking barefoot on contaminated floors or swimming pool decks and is nurtured by occlusive leather footwear.

Self-help treatment of athlete's foot is usually successful, and has three phases:

- Keep the feet well ventilated and dry. A daily shower is helpful, washing all areas carefully, including infection sites between the toes. Then dry thoroughly and wait ten minutes before donning shoes and socks. Cotton and wool socks should be worn instead of nylon; sandals and straw shoes are superior to leather.
- Attack the fungus infection with over-the-counter medication. A good old-fashioned remedy is iodochlorhydroxyquin (Vioform) cream applied three times daily. If using Vioform Cream, anticipate that nearby clothing may be stained yellow.
- A newer remedy is tolnaftate (Tinactin), available as a cream, solution, powder, or powder aerosol. Apply Tinactin twice daily for two or three weeks—until healing is complete.
- Once the feet are free of infection, recurrences can be prevented by applying zinc undecylenate/undecylenic acid (Desenex) spray or foot powder morning and evening.

Sometimes home treatment fails, and then successful therapy may require the doctor's prescription for griseofulvin (Grifulvin-V or Fulvicin) tablets to be taken once daily for up to eight weeks, plus professional local treatment.

Ringworm of the Scalp

The doctor calls it tinea capitis, but it's commonly known as scalp ringworm, and usually attacks youngsters. A patchy baldness appears, associated with itching and scaling of the scalp. Local treatment with tolnaftate (Tinactin) solution will subdue many cases of scalp ringworm, but the addition of prescription griseofulvin assures a much higher likelihood of successful treatment.

Ringworm of the Skin

No spot on the skin is immune from fungus infections, and I have seen them on the face, back, legs, and almost everywhere. Nevertheless, the fungus' favorite sites are warm, moist skin folds such as the groin, underarm, or folds under the breasts. When ringworm strikes these areas, there is redness, irritation, and itching.

Self-help treatment with tolnaftate (Tinactin) or iodochlorhydroxyquin (Vioform) cream applied two or three times daily will overcome most fungus infections of the skin. It's important to provide adequate ventilation, and lightweight, porous clothing should be worn.

In stubborn cases I have had success using ultraviolet phototherapy with the Spectroderm Lamp. In treating ringworm of the skin, as in other areas, a prescription for griseofulvin may be needed for widespread or resistant infections.

Fungus Infection of the Nail

Ringworm of the nails is called onychomycosis, and it's as difficult to treat as its name is to pronounce. The fungus-infected nail is thickened and distorted with irritation at the nailbed. In my opinion, no cream or ointment is worth two cents in the treatment of this deep-seated infection, and the only hope of eradicating onychomycosis is griseofulvin (Grifulvin V) tablets taken by prescription for at least six months when fingernails are infected and for at least 12 months to treat ringworm of the toenails.

GALLSTONES

Synonyms: gallbladder attack, cholelithiasis

At sometime during their lives, 15 percent of all men and 30 percent of all women develop gallstones. In many instances no symptoms occur and the stones are merely noted at autopsy. Yet in other individuals, stones in the gallbladder cause sufficient mischief to bring a patient to the operating table.

The gallbladder is a storage depot for bile, which forms in the liver, passes down the bile duct to be stored in the gallbladder, and is later released when needed in the intestine to dissolve fats. The entry of fats into the small intestine is the signal for the gallbladder to contract, forcing bile down the common bile duct into the small intestine.

During the time that bile is stored in the gallbladder, tiny crystals of cholesterol, bile pigments, and calcium sometimes form small stones (see Figure 14), which may subsequently grow, by a snowball effect, to form either a single gallstone as large as the gallbladder or up to two hundred tiny gallstones. Tiny stones are all the more dangerous since they may escape from the gallbladder and block the bile duct.

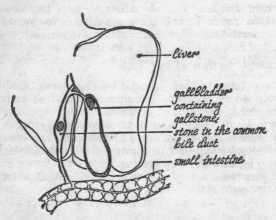

liver

gallbladder containing gallstone

stone in the common bile duct

small intestine

FIGURE 14. *Gallstones.*

When stones are present, contraction of the gallbladder forces the stone into the bladder opening, where it acts as a ball valve blocking the outflow of bile. The result is pain—the characteristic biliary colic with severe discomfort in the right upper quadrant of the abdomen. The pain may radiate to the upper back, and belching is common. Many times, gallbladder attacks subside spontaneously, although some show a stubborn resistance even to medical therapy and bring the patient to emergency surgery.

Avoiding and Treating the Gallbladder Attack

Since contraction of the gallbladder is stimulated by a fatty meal, gallbladder attacks are minimized by eating a diet low in fat and high in protein and carbohydrates. This means avoiding the following high-fat and gassy foods:

Pork	Duck
Mutton	Fried foods
Corned beef	Solid shortening
Fatty cuts of beef	Beans
Sausage	Cucumbers
Bacon	Cabbage
Ham	Radishes

A natural remedy that may relieve the acute gallbladder attack is a coffee enema. Brew a potful of strong natural coffee; decaffeinated or instant coffee won't do. Then mix one cupful of coffee to one pint of warm water and use as an enema held in the rectum for several minutes. Relief of the gallbladder attack often follows.

For an individual subject to gallbladder attacks (cholecystitis), the doctor will often prescribe an atropine-like medication such as propantheline (Pro-Banthine) to be taken every four to six hours as needed to relieve gallbladder spasm. Medication of this sort can be a lifesaver when, as often happens, the gallbladder attack occurs a few hours following the evening meal or even after retiring.

Surgery remains the definitive treatment for gallstones. Dissolving gallbladder calculi with medication (chenodesoxycholic acid) has received a recent flurry of publicity, but its general use is many years away; if, indeed, gallstone "dissolvers" ever prove to be of other than experimental interest.

131

Surgery is recommended for individuals with symptom-producing gallstones for the following reasons:

- Once a single gallbladder attack has been experienced, the probability is great that further attacks will occur.
- Subsequent gallbladder attacks may fail to subside spontaneously, and may progress to complications such as abscess or liver disease.
- Gallstones probably contribute to cancer of the gallbladder, admittedly an uncommon disease.
- Elective removal of the gallbladder (the only effective way to remove gallstones) allows surgery to be scheduled at a time convenient for patient and doctor. Why risk an emergency cholecystectomy in the middle of the night, with a sleepy surgeon operating on a dehydrated, exhausted patient who has failed to respond to medical treatment of his or her gallbladder attack?

GASTRITIS

Synonyms: heartburn, dyspepsia, acid stomach, acute indigestion

Anxiety, frustration, and dietary indiscretion combine to bring on gastritis—an acute inflammation of the stomach that causes a burning sensation in the upper abdomen and chest. Nervous tension plays a major role; and heartburn often follows an argument with the boss or spouse, an extra-hectic day at work, or any series of aggravating incidents. The gastritis sufferer is traditionally tense and conscientious, and drives himself beyond the tolerance of his stomach lining.

Food plays a major role, with coffee and alcohol prime precipitating factors, although most gastritis sufferers report that symptoms also follow spicy or acid foods, including tomatoes, fruit juices, pepperoni pizza, onions, and other tasty treats. Symptoms of gastritis are usually relieved by milk or by antacids that neutralize excessive acidity in the stomach.

Gastritis, which may be considered the first stage of a peptic ulcer, is most prevalent in the spring and fall of the year, although the reason for this seasonal variation is not known.

Medications may contribute to gastric irritation, and common offenders are aspirin, cortisone, phenylbutazone (Buta-zoladin), and indomethacin (Indocin).

Relieving Gastritis

When acid indigestion begins, it's time to ease tensions. Shun unnecessary responsibility and avoid aggravating situations, such as the maddening drive through downtown traffic and long hours of overtime at work. As a temporary crutch, the doctor may prescribe a mild tranquilizer such as chlordiazepoxide (Librium) or oxazepam (Serax).

Antacids neutralize stomach juices, and are available without prescription. They may be taken as often as every several hours, and can bring welcome relief when severe heartburn begins. Good choices include Riopan, Gelusil, and Maalox.

A bland diet helps rest the stomach lining. Eliminate spicy foods, coffee, and alcohol; instead the gastritis sufferer should take frequent small feedings of bland foods.

Bland Diet

Foods Permitted	Foods to Be Avoided
Cereals	
Cooked oat and wheat cereals	Dry precooked cereals
	Bran cereals
	Sugar-coated cereals
Breads	
White bread	Whole wheat bread
Muffins, rolls, and biscuits	
Corn bread	
Pancakes and waffles	
Soups	
Creamed soups	Bean, lentil, or split pea soups
Bouillon and broth	
Meat, Fish, and Dairy Products	
Boiled, baked, or broiled veal, ham, lean beef, turkey or chicken, and fish	Mutton and pork
	Fried or fatty meats
	Shellfish
Soft cooked eggs	Fried eggs
Cottage cheese	Cheese, except cottage cheese

133

Foods Permitted	Foods to Be Avoided

Vegetables

Carrots	Cucumbers
Lettuce	Brussels sprouts
Peas	Onions
Potatoes	Radishes
Spinach	Tomatoes
Corn	Cabbage
Beets	Squash
Celery	
Asparagus	
Green beans	

Fruits

Dilute fruit juices	Apples
Bananas	Apricots
Pears	Dates
Melons	Prunes
Plums	Oranges
Peaches	Rhubarb
	Pineapple
	Grapefruit
	Figs

Desserts

Cakes	Pies and pastries
Custard and pudding	Sherbet
Ice cream	
Gelatin	
Bread pudding	
Tapioca pudding	
Corn starch or rice pudding	

Beverages

Cocoa, Postum, and Ovaltine	Coffee, tea, and alcohol
Whole milk	Decaffeinated coffee
Skimmed milk	Carbonated beverages
	Buttermilk

Miscellaneous

Liquid vegetable oils (corn, soybean, and safflower)	Animal fats and lard
	Pepper
Sugar	Olives
Salt	Nuts
Macaroni and spaghetti	Pickles
Gravy	Tomato paste

Foods Permitted	Foods to Be Avoided
	Garlic
	Mayonnaise
	Mustard
	Horseradish
	Salted nuts
	Unsalted nuts
	Jelly and jam
	Relish
	Vinegar
	Candy
	Honey and molasses

When symptoms are severe, see the doctor. In addition to the measures described above, he may prescribe an anticholinergic medication such as propantheline (Pro-Banthine) or glycopyrrolate (Rubinul) to reduce acic formation in the stomach.

Almost all gastritis can be controlled by dietary changes and perhaps medication—if the patient follows the rules. The penalty for failure to treat gastritis may be the later development of a peptic ulcer (*q.v.*).

GLAUCOMA

Thousands of Americans over age 40 suffer glaucoma, an elevated fluid pressure within the eye that is a leading cause of blindness in older individuals. Early symptoms may be a vague discomfort within the eye, headache, or blurred vision with a rainbow or halo effect around lights, but often there are no complaints at all as pressure rises within the eye.

The diagnosis of glaucoma is confirmed upon finding fluid pressure in the eye above 20 mm of mercury when measured with a tonometer, and the doctor will recommend therapy to preserve vision.

Treating Glaucoma

Glaucoma therapy aims to reduce fluid pressure and to keep open the tiny channels that drain the aqueous humor from the anterior chamber of the eye. Often prescribed are pilocarpine eye drops, and perhaps a diuretic such as acetazolamide (Diamox).

Glaucoma victims must be wary of medications, since any drug with atropine-like side effects could aggravate glaucoma. These medications include belladonna, propantheline (Pro-Banthine) and many other medications prescribed for gastritis, peptic ulcer, irritable bowel, or diarrhea.

Glaucoma must be checked in the physician's office at regular intervals, because rising pressure (it can even happen during treatment) can cause permanent visual damage without producing pain.

To learn more about glaucoma, write to:

National Society for the Prevention of Blindness, Inc.
79 Madison Avenue
New York, New York 10016

Institute for Glaucoma Research
667 Madison Avenue
New York, New York 10021

GLOMERULONEPHRITIS

Synonym: nephritis

Like rheumatic fever, glomerulonephritis follows a streptococcal infection. Strep germs in the throat or on the skin provoke an inflammation of the kidney, causing dark, bloody urine, perhaps associated with headache, weakness, and flank pain. High blood pressure often occurs, and congestive heart failure may follow.

The microscopic finding of red blood cell casts in the urine is a tip-off, although the doctor may perform a needle biopsy of the kidney to confirm the diagnosis.

Treatment

There is no sure cure for glomerulonephritis. Therapy is directed toward symptoms: a lingering strep infection is treated with antibiotics such as penicillin. If high blood pressure is present, antihypertensive drugs are given. If fluid retention threatens to cause heart failure, a low-salt diet may be recommended.

Self-help treatment is to reduce salt and limit protein in the diet. Take fluids to flush waste products from the body, give yourself adequate rest, and avoid crowds where you may contract germs.

Glomerulonephritis usually subsides spontaneously over a period of weeks or months. In some individuals, a prolonged course is seen with continued presence of red blood cells in the urine. And a few unlucky victims suffer chronic glomerulonephritis, with impaired kidney function, protein in the urine, and the premature development of hypertension. For further information write:

National Kidney Foundation, Inc.
315 Park Avenue South
New York, New York 10010

GONORRHEA

Synonyms: "clap," drip, strain

The success of the sexual revolution has contributed to the rising incidence of gonorrhea, with an estimated two million new cases in the U.S. each year. Gonorrhea is a disease of the sexually active, and is most prevalent in the 15 to 24-year-old age group. Occurring 10 times more often than syphilis, gonorrhea is reported to afflict 10 to 33 percent of prostitutes.

Two to seven days following exposure, the male develops a thick creamy discharge from the penis, associated with frequent, painful urination, although some men suffer no discharge or discomfort. In the female, gonorrhea is often insidious, producing a profuse discharge of pus, but sometimes it causes only vague pelvic discomfort or perhaps no symptoms at all. Yet, in both men and women, persistent gonorrheal infections can cause permanent damage to reproductive organs and may result in sterility.

The Perils of Gonorrhea

Widespread though the epidemic of gonorrhea is known to be, individuals of both sexes and of all ages still decide to "take a chance." Here are facts that should be kept in mind:

- The "nice" girl or boy next door may be a gonorrhea carrier, as may the professional prostitute. In fact, the "pro" is likely to recognize and seek treatment for disease while the guilt-ridden youngster might conceal symptoms in the vain hope that they will go away.
- Don't count on prophylactic procedures. The condom offers some measure of protection but is far from foolproof. Scrubs, douches, and antibiotic ointments are of little value. The best prophylaxis is a firm "NO!"
- Self-treatment with a few leftover penicillin pills will almost certainly fail. Gonorrhea eradication requires large doses of antibiotics that should be administered under medical supervision.
- If you suspect gonorrhea, see the doctor. He'll check with a Thayer-Martin or Transgrow culture for a positive diagnosis. If gonorrhea is present, treatment should follow, using penicillin by injection, spectinomycin (Spectrocin) injection, or even with a single-dose liquid combination of ampicillin and probenecid (Polycillin-PBC). Following treatment, recheck cultures will be taken to confirm that the cure has been complete.
- Known or suspected sexual contacts of the patient with confirmed gonorrhea should have cultures taken. Only relentless follow-up can break the chain of gonorrheal infections and help stop the epidemic of this common venereal disease.

For further information write to:

American Social Health Association
1740 Broadway
New York, New York 10019

Center for Disease Control
Atlanta, Georgia 30333

GOUT

Synonym: gouty arthritis
The gout sufferer is in good company. Benjamin Franklin

suffered the disease, as did Francis Bacon, Michelangelo, Samuel Johnson, Charles Darwin, and Isaac Newton. In fact, the Stamp Act and the Tea Tax that led to the Boston Tea Party of 1773 were both passed by the British Parliament, despite William Pitt's well-known opposition to these acts, while Pitt was absent with the gout. Had William Pitt been healthy and present during the crucial sessions of Parliament, might the American Revolution never have occurred?

Gout is more common than generally supposed, affecting some 800,000 Americans. More than nine out of ten gout sufferers are males, and as Hippocrates observed in the fourth century B.C., "A woman does not take the gout, unless her menses be stopped."

Gout is a disorder of metabolism in which there are high blood levels of a compound called uric acid. Crystals of uric acid are deposited in joints, causing the characteristic heat, swelling, and intense pain. Commonly affected is the joint of the big toe, although other joints of the hands, arms, legs, and feet may be involved. Often an attack begins at night and may reach a peak within a few hours, lingering painfully for several days or more. Episodes may occur at long intervals of months or years, or may be separated by only a few weeks or days.

In time, deposits of uric acid may cause persistent joint swellings called tophi, and deposits of uric acid are sometimes also found on the external ear or in the kidneys. When high blood levels of uric acid go untreated, kidney stones may form.

Treatment

Dietary restrictions are a time-honored gout treatment. Although modern medication allows a more liberal diet than was once prescribed, the gout victim should avoid foods high in uric acid, including liver, sweetbreads, kidneys, herring, anchovies, sardines, shellfish, meat extracts, turkey, and beer.

Because uric acid crystals in the urine can form stones, it's a good idea to drink at least six to eight glasses of water daily.

Attacks of gout occur during times of stress, and gout therapy includes avoiding unaccustomed strenuous exercise, overexposure to cold, and inadequate rest.

Gout flare-ups often occur during times of tissue injury, including surgery. If you anticipate an operation or are under treatment for any serious illness, be sure that the physician is advised. He may wish to give medication to anticipate a gout attack.

Obesity aggravates gout, and it's best to maintain your ideal weight, although starvation diets must be avoided, since rapid tissue breakdown can also lead to an attack of gout.

Drug therapy gives gout the one-two punch: for the acute attack, the doctor will prescribe an anti-inflammatory drug such as colchicine, phenylbutazone (Butazoladin), oxyphenbutazone (Tandearil), indomethacin (Indocin), or cortisone. All share a tendency to cause gastrointestinal side effects and are usually prescribed for short-term use.

Once the acute attack of gout has subsided, prophylactic medicine is prescribed. The time-honored standard is probenecid (Benemid), although the physician may prescribe the newer allopurinol (Zyloprim).

Gout and drugs used to treat the disease are influenced by many medications, including aspirin, and individuals receiving drug therapy for gout should check with the physician before any other medication is taken.

The Outlook for Gout

Gout has been called the most treatable of all the rheumatic diseases. With careful follow-up, including blood tests and periodic adjustment of medication dosage, most gout victims today can be kept free of acute attacks. It requires diligence, the dietary restrictions mentioned above, and sensible health measures, but all who have experienced the excruciating pain of gout will agree that the effort is worthwhile.

Gout, classified as a type of arthritis, is discussed in pamphlets available from:

The Arthritis Foundation
1212 Avenue of the Americas
New York, New York 10036

HALITOSIS

Synonym: bad breath
Bad breath is a social handicap, an enemy of self-confi-

dence, and may signal the presence of disease in the mouth, throat, or chest. Think of halitosis not as a specific illness but as a symptom of many disorders, often disappearing when the cause is found and treated.

Bad Breath: Cause and Cure

Mouth-breathing causes morning breath, the arid taste of desert sand and cotton wool in the mouth upon arising. Often the culprit is nasal obstruction, and falling asleep is attended by eight hours of mouth-breathing that dries saliva and promotes oral infection. Bad breath responds to local mouthwash rinses (try Scope—it really helps), plus elimination of the nasal obstruction that forces nocturnal mouth-breathing.

Tooth and gum infections cause objectionable odors that result from decay and pus formation by bacteria. Antibiotics, rinses, and regular trips to the dentist often bring cure. Hidden disease in the nose or throat can cause halitosis, and possible causes include a chronic bacterial infection of the nose, infected adenoids, or a nasal polyp. Occasionally, a pocket in the back of the tongue collects food particles that disintegrate to form an objectionable odor; daily cleansing removes the debris and hence the halitosis.

Other potentially curable causes of bad breath include chronic sinus infection, chronic bronchitis, and an abscess of the lung.

In virtually all cases, the cure of halitosis awaits only diagnosis and treatment of the cause.

HANGOVER

Synonym: the morning after

Writing of New York City life in the Roaring Twenties, F. Scott Fitzgerald told: "The hangover became a part of the day as well allowed-for as the Spanish siesta."

The head pounds like a chorus of tympany, the eyes refuse to focus, and the teeth itch. Thoughts of food bring acute nausea, and a faltering hand reaches for "a hair of the dog that bit." What to do?

141

There's no sure cure, and perhaps this is as nature intended, for the hangover is just penance for the sins of the night before. The pounding headache will often respond to two aspirin, Bufferin, or acetaminophen (Tylenol) taken with a half glass of tepid water. An ice pack on the head helps bring relief, and, as the initial wave of nausea passes, soft bland foods may be taken, including toast, a poached egg, and warm beverage.

Coffee is an eye-opener, the strong aroma and caffeine content stimulating alertness. Some individuals who suffer frequent hangovers prefer caffeine pills, such as Nodoz Tablets containing 100 mg of caffeine (roughly equivalent to one cup of coffee).

Vitamins are a favorite remedy of hangover victims. They may have real value, or perhaps are merely placebos; no statistical study exists to document their benefits. For what they're worth, the following are favorite over-the-counter remedies:

- Chaser for Hangover, containing caffeine, niacinamide, thiamine, oil of peppermint, acetaminophen, aspirin, plus aluminum and magnesium buffers.
- Tirend Tablets containing niacin, thiamine, dextrose, and caffeine.

The doctor may offer whiffs of oxygen and/or inject 25 mg of thiamine to prevent complications of chronic and acute alcohol ingestion.

All of the above remedies will be unnecessary, if those who enjoy alcoholic beverages practice moderation in imbibing.

HAY FEVER

Synonyms: allergic rhinitis, pollen allergy

"Hay fever" describes a host of ills, with symptoms of sneezing, watery eyes, itching of the nose, sinus congestion, and cough. The cause is pollen allergy, and because symptoms are most prevalent during autumn when hay is harvested the malady has long been called hay fever—stigmatizing this hapless animal fodder—when the real culprit is airborne pollen of ragweed and other weeds.

Similar symptoms appear in the spring, caused by grass and tree pollens. At this time the disease may be called rose fever, another misnomer, since the rose's only connection with allergic rhinitis is that it blooms when the patient's symptoms are most intense.

Treatment

Self-help medical treatment involves avoiding pollens and alleviating symptoms. When ragweed pollen is at its peak between mid-August and late September, the sufferer would be best advised to take a month-long ocean voyage. However, since this is rarely practical, certain household precautions will minimize respiratory symptoms until the first frost lowers airborne pollen pollution.

Air conditioning helps immeasurably, by filtering air entering the house and by removing excessive humidity. Room air-conditioning units are okay; central air conditioning is better (and a tax-deductible medical expense if prescribed by the physician). Don't neglect to clean the air filter regularly.

Household dust and pollen catchers should be eliminated. This includes fluffy carpets, frilly draperies, open bookcases, and nicknacks that trap airborne particles. Dust the house each day with a damp cloth to keep allergenic substances to a minimum.

An electrostatic air filter can be a lifesaver in early autumn, eliminating circulating pollens in household air. Be sure it is cleaned monthly, not only to ensure that it functions properly but to avoid the possibility that sparks will cause fire if the grid becomes caked with dust and dirt.

The hay fever victim soon learns that Labor Day is no time for a picnic in the meadow, and he wisely leaves autumn grass-cutting to a neighborhood youngster.

The local pharmacy abounds with over-the-counter medication to relieve hay fever, rose fever, and other types of allergic rhinitis. Available are antihistamines, decongestants, a vast array of combination antihistamine-decongestant tablets and capsules, and nasal sprays to open plugged noses.

Inhiston, which has been my mother's cure-all for nasal

143

congestion for as long as I can remember, contains the antihistamine pheniramine maleate.

Most potent of the pure decongestants is Sudafed, available as a 30-mg tablet of pseudoephedrine. Sixty-milligram Sudafed Tablets are often prescribed by doctors; the same medication is available without prescription and without an office call simply by using two 30-mg Sudafed Tablets.

Of the many combination antihistamine-decongestants available, the following are my first choices in the non-prescription treatment of hay fever:

- Contac Capsules, containing phenylpropanolamine, chlorpheniramine, and a drying belladonna alkaloid—all packed in a time-disintegration capsule.
- Dristan Twelve-hour Decongestant Capsules containing chlorpheniramine and phenylephrine.
- Coricidin-D Decongestant Tablets containg phenylephrine, chlorpheniramine, caffeine, and aspirin.

Decongestant nasal sprays often bring more relief than pills and can be safely used in conjunction with antihistamine-decongestant combinations. Two sprays in each nostril help reduce swollen nasal membranes and minimize secretions. Be wary, since excessive use can foster dependency upon the product and cause a "rebound" congestion when use of the spray is discontinued. Nasal sprays are for occasional use only. Of the more than one dozen possible choices, my favorites are:

- Afrin Nasal Spray, containing oxymetazoline hydrochloride, the most potent topical decongestant available with or without a prescription. Spray twice in each nostril every twelve hours; no more.
- Neo-Synephrine Nasal Spray containing phenylephrine hydrochloride, and available in 0.25 and 0.50-percent solutions.

What the Doctor Can Do

When you've tried, you've *really tried*, to avoid airborne pollens, and you've sampled every pill and nasal spray the pharmacy has to offer, yet sneezing and nasal congestion persist; then it's time to call the doctor.

The physician may prescribe therapeutic doses of a pure antihistamine such as chlorpheniramine (Chlor-Trimeton) or tripelennamine (Pyribenzamine). Or he may write a prescription for a stronger decongestant-antihistamine combination, perhaps Ornade Spansule Capsules containing chlorpheniramine, phenylpropanolamine hydrochloride, and isopropamide as a drying agent. At best these preparations offer relief of symptoms, and there's an increased risk of the drowsiness common to all antihistamine preparations.

When and if symptomatic treatment with antihistamine and/or decongestant preparations fails, the doctor may advise a short course of cortisone treatment, particularly if symptoms are expected to last only another few weeks. A common prescription is prednisone tablets taken three or four times daily for one to two weeks, tapering off over the last few days. Relief is dramatic, and short-term treatment usually avoids the formidable hazards of long-term cortisone therapy.

Often the doctor's advice is for desensitization therapy—allergy shots to build immunity to offending pollens, molds, or whatever the cause of the allergy. Shots begin once or twice weekly, eventually becoming less frequent, perhaps as long as a month apart. Most highly allergic individuals receiving desensitization report good results, with relative freedom from symptoms during the hay fever season.

For further information write to:

Allergy Foundation of America
801 Second Avenue
New York, New York 10017

National Institute of Allergy and Infectious Disease
Information Office
Bethesda, Maryland 20014

HEAD TRAUMA

Synonyms: head injury, blow to the head, concussion

A fall from a horse, an encounter with a mugger, a two-car accident—all are likely causes of head trauma. How to tell the severity of the injury? Has brain damage occurred? Should you call the doctor?

Few head injuries develop serious problems, a comforting fact to remember when your son's head encounters a thrown rock or flying baseball bat. Most victims suffer severe local pain, perhaps attended by a brief dazed period, then recover uneventfully without treatment. But a few are not so lucky, and head injuries are assessed in an attempt to determine those individuals in need of further therapy.

Unconsciousness is a dangerous symptom, and many hospital emergency rooms categorically admit for observation all individuals suffering unconsciousness (however brief) associated with head trauma.

Another ominous sign is repeated forceful vomiting, described as "projectile." Following head trauma, youngsters cry vigorously, swallowing mucus and tears; then there's the hysteria of onlookers and relatives, perhaps complicated by a hurried trip to the doctor. Small wonder that the upset child vomits once or even twice. But repeated and extra-forceful vomiting may signal brain injury and deserves medical evaluation.

Increasing lethargy is another worrisome symptom, and the head trauma victim who shows progressive drowsiness should be taken to the doctor.

A headache is expected, and local discomfort following head injury should be treated with ice packs. However, a headache that increases days or weeks after a head injury should be suspect.

How about skull fractures? Certainly a cracked cranium signals a more severe injury than a simple bruise, but remember that it's damage to the brain (not the skullbone) that causes worry. Two types of skull fractures are found: the first is a linear fracture, like a single crack in an eggshell. Nothing is out of place, and the crack will mend without treatment. More ominous is the depressed skull fracture, with a fragment of skull pushed inward toward the brain. Here the potential for brain damage is high, and surgery is often recommended to elevate the fracture fragment. Nevertheless, x-rays fail to tell the whole story and bleeding within the brain may occur with a perfectly intact skull.

Most head injuries are treated with "observation," and here is a list of instructions that doctors have found useful:

Although examination reveals no evidence of serious injury, complications may become evident later. The doctor should be called immediately, no matter what the hour, if any of the following occur:

- Vomiting, either repeated or forceful.
- A stiff neck, which causes pain with attempts at forward flexion.
- Convulsive seizure or epileptic fit.
- Inappropriate behavior or delirium.
- One pupil (the black center of the eye) larger than the other.
- Weakness of an arm or leg.
- Blood or clear fluid draining from the nose or ear.
- Headache that increases in severity.
- Unexpected drowsiness, or difficulty in awakening the patient.
- Any other symptom that seems unusual or causes you to worry.

During the first 24 hours the patient should be observed every two to four hours, night and day. The patient or family should keep the doctor's telephone number handy, ready to call promptly if even one of these symptoms are noted following a head injury.

HEADACHE

Synonym: cephalgia

There are more types of headaches than you have fingers to count them. Headache may accompany fever or sinus infection, and is the hallmark of a viral flu. Fluid retention can cause a pressure type of headache seen a few days before a woman's menstrual period, or on the morning after a bout of heavy drinking. Sometimes a dull frontal headache follows sleeping in a poorly ventilated room or smoking too many cigarettes the night before. There are persons who insist that constipation causes headaches and others whose cephalgia is blamed upon eye strain, bright lights, an overheated room, or working in poor illumination. Sometimes headache follows the use of medication (notably vasodilators such as nitroglycerin) or is caused by high blood pressure. And, a concern of many cephalgia suffers, an occasional headache is due to a tumor of the brain.

Of most interest are the vascular headache syndromes—the classic causes of cephalgia—responsible for most chronic headache problems. Common to these syndromes is headache pain that follows the opening up (dilation) of small blood vessels within the skull. When tiny arteries and/or veins open, pressure within the cranium increases—and pain results.

Cluster headaches, also called histamine headaches, are uncommon, but afflicted individuals are quick to point out that their relative rarity is overshadowed by their being the most painful of the headache syndromes. Headache episodes occur about once daily for three or four weeks, then disappear for months or years—hence the name cluster headache. The usual pain is one-sided, begins abruptly, rapidly reaches a peak, then subsides after about an hour. The eye on the involved side is red, and there is one-sided nasal stuffiness. Because of the short duration of cephalgia, analgesics usually are of little value; by the time medication is absorbed, the headache has already begun to wane.

Many cluster headache sufferers have recognized that their episodes begin when tension rises. I recall one medical school professor who personally suffered with the histamine headache syndrome and said, "When I start to have my headaches, I know it's time for a vacation." Adequate emotional and physical rest may be prophylactic, as might be avoidance of alcohol, since some histamine headache sufferers find their attacks triggered by alcohol ingestion. In addition, it sometimes helps to avoid high-serotonin foods, including wine (especially red wine), liver, and cheddar cheese. The doctor may prescribe prophylactic medication such as ergotamine (Gynergen), cyproheptadine (Periactin), or methylsergide (Sansert).

Migraine headache is also one-sided. Often preceded by an aura of spots before the eyes or visual distortion, the migraine headache reaches its peak more slowly then the histamine headache, and lasts longer—often four hours or more. Nausea and vomiting are not uncommon, and the patient is incapacitated until the cephalgia is relieved. Ice packs on the head may help, as may aspirin or acetaminophen (Tylenol).

One novel treatment is reported to bring relief to two-thirds of migraine headache sufferers: Sit under a hair dryer when headache pain occurs; the dryer's warmth and high-pitched hum relax tension and help banish pain. Yet these measures are usually inadequate, and the doctor often prescribes an ergotamine preparation to combat the wide-open arteries causing increased pressure within the cranium. Stronger analgesics such as propoxyphene (Darvon), or codeine may be prescribed, as may be prophylactic daily doses of methylsergide maleate (Sansert).

Tension headache is by far the most common of all headache syndromes. The pain is less intense than with histamine or migraine headaches, and usually builds up more gradually (see Figure 15). Usually found in the temples or across the forehead, the pain of tension headache often follows concentrated effort, sustained anxiety, or chronic aggravation. Specific treatment includes reduction of tension-producing responsibilities, an increased allotment of stress-free recreation, and pain relief using simple analgesics such as aspirin, acetaminophen (Tylenol) or propoxyphene (Darvon), occasionally supplemented by the prescription for a mild tranquilizer such as chlordiazepoxide (Librium).

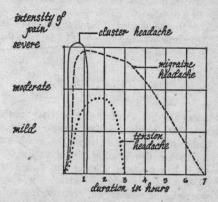

FIGURE 15. *Comparison of pain and duration of cluster, migraine, and tension headaches.*

Some factors contribute to many types of headache. It makes good sense to follow these ten rules:

- Avoid overwork and excessive emotional tension. Sidestep needless responsibility whenever possible.
- Keep your schedule regular and unhurried, and allow for at least eight hours sleep each night.
- Avoid prolonged eye strain, and be sure not to work in glaring or inadequate light.
- Shun the din of excessive noise that can cause headache pain.
- Stay out of stuffy overheated rooms.
- Don't smoke and avoid rooms full of smokers.
- Take no alcoholic beverages, since they may trigger some headache syndromes.
- If headaches are one-sided and quite severe (such as cluster or migraine cephalgia), avoid high-serotonin foods including red wine, cheddar cheese, liver, and sausage.
- Take frequent short vacations to get away from the strain of work.
- Check with the doctor if headaches don't respond to self-help remedies, and follow his advice to the letter.

HEART ATTACK

Synonyms: myocardial infarction, coronary occlusion

An estimated half million Americans suffer heart attacks each year, and more than one-quarter of these victims die, making heart disease the leading single cause of death in America. And unless medical science can find some way to end the trend, deaths due to heart attacks will continue to rise as our overfed, underexercised, frenetic life style leads to increasing coronary atherosclerosis. (For a further discussion of self-help prevention of atherosclerosis, see page 37.)

To discuss a heart attack, and to understand what the doctor may tell you, it's necessary to know some definitions. "Coronary" is an adjective referring to the heart; coronary arteries are tiny arteries supplying the heart muscle. The heart muscle, called the myocardium, supplies the forceful push of heart contraction, and may be damaged or even suffer "death" of a small section when its blood supply is compromised. The correct term for this phenomenon is "infarction," meaning death of tissue following impairment of its blood supply. "Occlusion" means a blockage, and thus a coronary occlusion means a blockage in the small arteries of the heart.

Let's put it all together: A heart attack is a coronary occlusion (blockage of the small arteries to the heart) causing an infarction (tissue death due to poor blood supply of the myocardial muscle of the heart wall).

Heart attacks strike the same individuals subject to angina (q.v.): the fat person, the heavy smoker, the carrier of high blood cholesterol and fat, the hypertensive, and the frantic high producer whose responsibilities keep him running full speed all day long.

The symptoms of heart attack may mimic angina, with a chest pain radiating down the left arm; but they usually differ by being more severe and "crushing" than angina, poorly responsive to nitroglycerin, and often associated with pallor, shortness of breath, and prostration. Here's one tip-off to the diagnosis: the heart attack victim often describes his pain by clenching his fist to the chest. But don't be fooled: many heart attacks are "silent" or nearly so, causing misleading symptoms such as upper abdominal pain, discomfort in the jaw, aching in the shoulder and head, "gas" pain, or a vague sensation of chest tightness. If any of these symptoms occur, call the physician at once.

Sometimes the onset is dramatic, and the heart attack victim suffers sudden shock with labored breathing. If you are on the scene, begin resuscitation (see page 263) if necessary, discourage onlookers from administering nitroglycerin, coffee, or stimulants, give oxygen by mask as soon as it's available (perhaps the police car carries an oxygen tank), keep the patient reclining and covered with a blanket, and summon the ambulance urgently.

In the Hospital

In-hospital treatment of a heart attack varies according to the severity of the attack, but certain basic patterns emerge.

Bed rest will be enforced, at least during the first few days, and the heartbeat will be monitored electronically while electrocardiograms and blood tests confirm the diagnosis of a heart attack. If pain is present, morphine or meperidine (Demerol) may be administered, and intravenous lidocaine may be given to prevent or suppress an irregular heart rhythm. To prevent blood clots and their complications, the doctor may "thin out the blood" with an anticoagulant such as heparin or warfarin (Coumadin). Oxygen may be given if shortness of breath is present, and the doctor will prescribe sedatives, a diuretic, and other medication as needed.

Initial treatment will be given in the coronary care unit—a speicalized treatment area where heart attack and other high-risk patients are gathered, and where the most modern electronic devices are found, plus highly trained nurses who can act independently in emergencies. After five to ten days of therapy in the coronary care unit, the heart attack victim is moved to a regular hospital bed. The doctor will supervise gradual resumption of activities—sitting on the edge of the bed, up in a chair, standing, then walking down the hall. Oh, how the patient celebrates these little triumphs.

At the end of three to four weeks of hospitalization, it's out the door and home. But rest continues even there. Prescribed may be an afternoon nap, avoidance of stairs, and a limitation on the number of visitors. During the next few months household activities increase with added chores, short outdoor walks, drives in the car, and visits to church and social functions.

Finally, about three to four months following the initial heart attack, the doctor may give his okay to return to work.

Preventing Heart Attacks

Here are some tips to help prevent your first heart attack, or to avoid a recurrence following recovery from a myocardial infarction:

- Stay slim. Adiposity adds an unnecessary strain to the heart's function, and weight loss can ease the circulatory burden.
- Don't smoke, since nicotine compromises blood flow to the heart muscle.
- Treat hypertension vigorously; poorly controlled high

blood pressure is a frequent forerunner of a coronary occlusion.

- Stabilize blood cholesterol and fat levels. This means a trip to the doctor for blood lipid analysis, perhaps followed by dietary changes or medication. High blood lipid levels increase the risk of coronary occlusion, and a cholesterol level over 250 mg carries twice the risk of coronary heart disease as a cholesterol level below 220 mg per 100 ml.
- Exercise daily, strengthening the muscles while increasing the heart's exercise tolerance. Begin gradually, then augment the exercise program as strength and stamina grow. A first-rate exercise program is found on page 39.
- If you are a high-risk patient, or have suffered a previous heart attack, see the doctor regularly. He may prescribe anticoagulants or other medication, and he'll certainly want to check your weight and blood pressure at frequent internals. Keep your appointments and follow his advice, and you will increase the odds of avoiding a heart attack.
- Read *The Heart Doctor's Heart Book* by Marshall Franklin, Martin Krauthamer, A. R. Tai, and Ann Pinchot (Grosset & Dunlap, New York), stressing prevention with specific recommendations for the cardiac patient.

If you're interested in learning more about heart attacks and how they can be prevented, request information from:

The American Heart Association, Inc.
7320 Greenville Avenue
Dallas, Texas 75231

You might ask for one or more of the following booklets:

The Way to a Man's Heart (a fat-controlled, low-cholesterol meal plan)
Smoking and Heart Disease
The Heart and Blood Vessels
After a Coronary

HEART FAILURE

Synonym: congestive heart failure

The heart never rests, but beats day and night to maintain circulation of the blood and carry vital nutrients to all organs of the body. The heart rate increases with exercise and slows with rest, but the heart never stops until life's end.

Blood coming to the heart through the veins is oxygen-poor and laden with carbon dioxide wastes. The right chambers of the heart pump the blood through the lungs, where wastes are discharged and life-giving oxygen is taken up. Next the blood returns to the heart, where the next beat sends it pulsing through the great aorta and thence to arteries throughout the body. As blood passes through the heart, its one-way journey is assured by a series of four valves within the heart that prevent the backflow of this life-stustaining fluid.

What then is "congestive heart failure"? It's simply the failure of the heart to pump blood out as fast as it arrives at the heart. When this happens, blood backs up in the lungs, where congestion causes shortness of breath most noticeable when reclining. Swollen ankles develop due to the combined effects of back pressure in the veins and gravity. As the fluid content of blood backs up in the tissues, body weight increases, and lung congestion often prohibits sleeping flat at night.

Controlling Congestive Heart Failure

When swollen ankles and nocturnal shortness of breath occur, a date with the doctor is mandatory. Following tests, he will probably prescribe digitalis (a favorite brand is Lanoxin) and/or a fluid-eliminating diuretic (of the many brands available, favorites include Diuril, Esidrex, Dyazide, Hygroton, or Aldactizide).

But medication is only part of the treatment. Equally important are self-help efforts that can assist in controlling congestive failure:

- Elevating the head of the bed at night helps prevent fluid accumulation in the lungs. The number of pillows necessary for easy breathing is a gauge of severity of the heart failure and a good guide to the success of treatment.

- Rest daily, including a mid-morning and mid-after-noon session off your feet with the legs elevated. This reduces the strain on the heart, and returns swollen ankle fluid to the body where it can be eliminated via the kidneys.
- Don't smoke!
- Reduce your salt intake, since salt increases the blood's fluid content and adds a strain on the heart. The doctor may prescribe a rigid salt-free regimen, but often it's not necessary to buy expensive salt-free foods. All that's needed is hiding the salt shaker, plus avoidance of inherently high-salt foods such as:

> Meat stock soups and bouillon
> Most canned vegetables
> Sauerkraut
> Bacon
> Corned beef
> Ham
> Salt fish
> Sausage
> Shellfish
> Whole milk and cream
> Salted nuts, popcorn, or potato chips
> Mustard and horseradish
> Olives and pickles
> Monosodium glutamate

- Some medicines, such as sodium salicylate that may be taken for arthritis, are extra-high in sodium, and overuse may negate the efforts of diuretics and salt restriction. Other drugs, such as thyroid medication and some diet pills, add an extra burden to the heart's efforts. Before taking any medication, the individual with congestive heart failure should ask the physician, "Will this affect my heart?"
- As improvement occurs, there will be a weight loss due to fluid elimination. Record the weight daily at the same time and wearing the same clothes or pajamas (or nothing). A gradual weight decline shows the success of initial therapy and a stable weight indi-

cates that congestive heart failure is well controlled. On the other hand, a sudden gain in weight may signal worsening of the heart failure and may precede more severe symptoms such as acute shortness of breath.

With continued improvement, shortness of breath disappears, ankle swelling leaves, and once again there is restful sleep with only one pillow. At this time the physician may give his approval to graded exercise beginning with walking, perhaps eventually progressing to the conditioning exercises described on page 39.

HEAT RASH

Synonyms: prickly heat, miliaria

Heat rash can often be traced to hot, humid weather and heavy occlusive clothing. Called miliaria by physicians, heat rash is an inflammation of the sweat glands seen as multiple tiny red bumps on the skin. Most often involved are the neck, beltline, and diaper area.

Treatment

Air conditionng and light clothing help, and may be all that's needed for mild cases. Periodic sponging of affected areas with cool water helps relieve symptoms and, after drying, irritated areas may respond to a talcum dusting powder such as good old Johnson's Baby Powder.

An excellent prickly heat remedy is a cool colloidal oatmeal (Aveeno) bath. Inflamed areas may respond to applications of sap of the Aloe Vera plant; break the stem of this tropical plant and apply the watery gel directly to the heat rash, or buy the commercial preparation called Alo-Creme.

HEMOPHILIA

A sex-linked recessive trait, hemophilia is carried by females and affects only males. The disorder was described in the early Jewish Talmud and circumcision was proscribed in families who suffered this disorder. In later years, the occurrence of hemophilia in royal families of the Continent, especially Russia, brought worldwide attention to the disorder.

Hemophilia is a defect of Factor VIII, needed for blood clotting. Bleeding episodes occur, most troublesome when they strike vital organs or major joints.

Information concerning home care, medical therapy and possible available funds may be obtained from these sources:

National Hemophilia Foundation
25 West 39th Street
New York, New York 10018

National Genetics Foundation
250 West 57th Street
New York, New York 10019

National Foundation—March of Dimes
P. O. Box 2000
White Plains, New York 10602

HEMORRHOIDS

Synonym: piles

Hemorrhoids are varicose veins around the rectum, and like varicose veins of the legs, may accompany underactivity that allows blood to pool in these venous channels. Inflammation often occurs, and hemorrhoids may enlarge following diarrhea, constipation, or straining at stool. A thrombosed hemorrhoid contains a blood clot, which often occurs suddenly, seen and felt as a discrete blue-purple enlargement like a grape hanging from the anal area.

Treatment

Most cases of mild hemorrhoids can be treated at home. Heat relieves acute inflammation, and it helps to sit in a tub of hot water (elegantly called a sitz bath) for one-half hour three times daily; be sure to elevate your bottom from the floor of the tub so that the warm water can exert its healing action on the hemorrhoidal tissues. If a tub bath is impractical, moist heat can be applied with a hot, damp cloth, applied to the rectum for 30 minutes three times daily.

Witch hazel helps shrink hemorrhoids, and a sitz bath may be followed by an application of witch hazel for a few minutes after drying. Equally effective, and quite handy, are Tucks—throwaway cotton flannel pads impregnated with glycerine and witch hazel. Tucks may also be used instead of toilet paper to wipe following a bowel movement.

Many soothing hemorrhoidal ointments are available without prescription and two good choices are:

- Medicone Rectal Unguent containing benzocaine, oxyquinolone, menthol, zinc oxide, petrolatum, lanolin, and Balsam Peru.
- Anusol Hemorrhoidal Ointment, which contains benzyl benzoate, bismuth subgallate, bismuth resorcin compound, Balsam Peru, zinc oxide, boric acid, and cocoa butter.

A good home remedy for hemorrhoids is insertion of a suppository made of raw potato. It's soothing, astringent, and often brings dramatic relief.

Hemorrhoids that fail to respond to self-help therapy, those that bleed, and recurrent piles should be treated by the physician. Perhaps he will prescribe a preparation containing cortisone, such as Wyanoid-HC Suppositories or Anusol HC Cream. Severe recurrent hemorrhoids are often removed surgically.

Hemorrhoid Prevention

One prevention tip can be better than a dozen clever cures, and hemorrhoids can often be avoided by wiping the anal area gently, plus taking plenty of bran and natural roughage in the diet (see page 72). Constipation and diarrhea must be avoided; don't hesitate to use a dose or two of milk of magnesia or Kaopectate as needed. Finally, you should avoid prolonged sitting or standing that can allow blood to pool in painful hemorrhoids.

HEPATITIS

Synonyms: viral hepatitis, jaundice

Hepatitis is an inflammation of the liver—the large abdominal organ that regulates much of the body's chemistry and produces bile to aid in the absorption of fats. Symptoms of viral hepatitis include a loss of appetite, achiness, and fatigue, plus a telltale yellow color (jaundice) of the skin and eyes.

Two types of viral hepatitis are known: Hepatitis A (also called infectious hepatitis or epidemic hepatitis) is most commonly carried in the stool and acquired by oral ingestion via contaminated food, drink, utensils, cigarettes, "joints," and so forth.

Hepatitis B (previously called serum hepatitis, transfusion hepatitis, or homologous serum jaundice) is chiefly spread through innoculation of blood or blood products from infected donors, but recent evidence has shown that the disease can be spread by other means, including sexual contact. Doctors detect the presence of hepatitis B by a blood test for the hepatitis B antigen (previously called the Australia antigen), which persists even after the liver inflammation has subsided, and is present in 0.08 to 0.26 percent of apparently healthy individuals.

Both hepatitis A and B cause similar symptoms, although the incubation period of hepatitis Type A (two to six weeks) is somewhat shorter than that of Type B (six weeks to six months). With either disease, the patient may complain of fever, weakness, malaise, headache, loss of appetite, and jaundice; the treatment of both types is the same.

Treatment

No specific therapy is available for hepatitis, and the physician will usually recommend supportive measures, including rest, diet, and supplementary vitamins. Rest in bed, perhaps at home or in the hospital, is advised during the active stages of disease. Even household chores exert a metabolic strain on the liver and should be avoided while jaundice is acute. As symptoms begin to subside, limited activity within the household is permitted, but work is undertaken only with the doctor's permission.

A nutritious diet is advised. Through the centuries of history, doctors have advised this diet or that for the treatment of jaundice. Some were high in protein, some high in carbohydrates, and some patently foolish. Today we know that the patient need only eat a nutritious balanced diet, catering to the reduced appetite often found in hepatitis victims.

Supplementary vitamins are often advised, since the intake of vital nutrients may be impaired by a lagging appetite. One good choice is Optilet M-500 Vitamins, one tablet taken twice daily.

It has been my own observation that sunbathing helps reduce jaundice of the skin although this probably has little or no effect on the basic liver disease.

Rest and isolation are continued until the doctor says, "Your blood tests are now back to normal. You can resume your usual activities as long as there is no consumption of alcohol or exposure to potentially harmful chemicals."

Preventing the Spread of Hepatitis

Hepatitis A, and to some extent Type B, is spread by personal contact, tainted food, and contaminated objects. Scrupulous cleanliness is needed to prevent transmission to other members of the household. This calls for isolation of the hepatitis patient's utensils and dishes (paper plates and plastic utensils are a good bet), towels, and linen. The patient and his attendants should scrub their hands frequently, and paper towels are advised. Ideally, the hepatitis patient has a separate bathroom, and this should receive a thorough cleansing with a disinfectant each day.

Gamma globulin injections are advised for household members in contact with patients suffering hepatitis A, and is particularly intended for those persons who shared food with the infected individual. Although not foolproof, gamma globulin administration has proved to be a most effective prophylaxis when given to the hepatitis-exposed individual. Gamma globulin injections are also recommended for travelers departing for high-risk hepatitis areas of the world.

HERNIA

Synonym: "strain"

The hernia begins as a weak spot in the muscular wall of the abdomen; with a cough or sneeze, the abdominal lining (peritoneum) and sometimes the bowel balloon out to lie directly beneath the skin. Although the groin (inguinal) hernia is most common, hernias may occur at other areas, such as the navel or the femoral area of the upper thigh.

Inguinal Hernia

The inguinal hernia protrudes through a ring in the lower abdominal wall. Many a youngster is born with an inguinal hernia or develops one shortly after birth. When found, an infant's hernia should be repaired promptly, since these show a distressing tendency to become trapped and block the bowel.

The adult hernia often begins when forceful straining exceeds the tolerance of a previously existing weak spot in the supporting tissues. A sudden painful "pop" may be noted, followed by a persistent or recurrent bulge that transmits the impulse of coughing.

Surgical correction is advised in almost all cases, since hernias don't subside, but rather tend to become larger and larger. A truss, once a favored hernia remedy, should be used rarely today, perhaps to temporize until a convenient surgical date or for individuals too elderly or infirm for surgery.

Umbilical Hernia

The umbilical hernia is a common occurrence in young infants and occurs when there is an opening in the muscular wall beneath the navel. As crying increases abdominal pressure, the hernia protrudes to look like a small sausage appended to the abdomen. Most umbilical hernias subside before the age of two years, and efforts to "hold in the hernia" with adhesive tape are futile, and often succeed only in causing an adhesive-tape dermatitis.

An umbilical hernia that fails to subside during infancy

can be corrected surgically, as can the occasional umbilical hernia occurring in an adult.

Femoral Hernia

The femoral hernia is much like the umbilical hernia, but pops out below the inguinal ligament and thus is found beneath the groin crease. Often occurring in women, the femoral hernia transmits the impulse of coughing and is most noticeable upon standing. Surgery is the only reliable treatment and is recommended for all individuals who are deemed good surgical candidates.

HERPES VIRUS INFECTION

Synonyms: cold sore, fever blister, herpes simplex infection, herpes progenitalis

The ubiquitous cold sore has been called "the most widespread pathogen of man" and can affect not only the lips and mouth, but the eyes, urinary membranes, intestinal organs, respiratory tissues, and genital organs. Doctors now report that herpes simplex infection is the second most common venereal disease among young Americans and is suspected of causing cancer of the cervix.

The cold sore is caused by herpes virus hominis, which lives in the tissues, bursting into bloom when the body's defenses are lowered by a common cold, flu, sunburn, menstrual period, pregnancy, or any factor that alters metabolism. Then tiny blisters develop, which progress to form a crusted, swollen, painful skin infection. The "fever blister" infection characteristically lasts for 10 to 14 days, then subsides, only to recur again a few weeks or months later.

Treatment

Traditional therapy has been disappointing. Over the centuries practically every topical medicine known to mankind has been applied to fever blisters, including alcohol, ether, tincture of benzoin, Bacitracin Ointment, etc. Although these measures may prevent secondary bacterial infection in some cases, they have failed to alter the course of the herpes simplex infection.

During the past few years, a new, possibly effective, but somewhat controversial treatment has been used. It's called the dye-light treatment and should begin when the first symptoms develop. Tiny blisters are opened gently using a sterile needle and any scabs are removed. The cold sore is painted with a 0.1-percent aqueous solution of proflavine sulfate dye. After an interval of six to eight hours, the cold sore is irradiated using an ordinary fluorescent-lamp tube (from a desk lamp, for example), for 30 minutes at a distance of about four inches, repeating the procedure 24 hours later. If the cold sore is attacked early in its course, the lesion is dry and healing within about three days.

The dye-light treatment works by photosensitization, allowing the light to break down the herpes virus, and rendering the viral particles noninfectious.

But there's a catch. Some physicians claim that the dye-light treatment may prove harmful, citing evidence that photo-inactivated viruses cause cancer-like changes in tissue culture cells, and they urge caution. And scientific studies in 1976 suggested that the dye-light treatment may have no more than placebo effect.

A useful and certainly safer self-help remedy is as follows: Break the blisters with an alcohol-cleansed needle, then apply talc—ordinary talcum powder—and leave open to the air. Repeat the application four times daily until the herpes virus infection has cleared.

HICCUPS

The hiccup is a rhythmic contraction of the diaphragm—the large muscle separating chest and abdomen. Often simple hiccups follow distention (overstretching) of the abdomen; or the diaphragm may undergo rhythmic spasm without apparent cause.

Mercifully, hiccups are usually short-lived. Many remedies have been devised, and objective evaluation of their efficacy is hampered by the self-limited nature of hiccups. But for what they are worth, here are six handy hiccup remedies:

- Hold the breath as long as possible, while straining against the closed glottis (throat). This time-honored treatment combats muscular spasm of the diaphragm and aborts most hiccups. The maneuver also alters the blood pressure and strains the heart mómentarily; it's not recommended if you suffer or suspect heart disease.
- Rebreathe carbon dioxide from a paper bag held over the face. It sounds silly, but often works.
- Attempt drinking a glass of water while a pencil is held clenched in the teeth. (Wear old clothes.)
- Hold the tongue outstretched for three minutes.
- Induce nausea by holding the finger down the throat.
- Take one teaspoonful of syrup of ipecac—this will be followed by nausea and perhaps vomiting.

If all else fails and hiccups seem destined to last forever, call the doctor, who may suggest whiffs of ether or perhaps an injection of diazepam (Valium).

HIVES

Synonym: urticaria

Hives are welts occurring anywhere on the body, and often subsiding as quickly as they appear—only to arise elsewhere. Most hives are caused by allergy, although anxiety is a cause of some cases of chronic urticaria. When allergy is the cause, the offending substance has usually been taken by mouth as food, drink, or medication, although other possible causes include injections (such as penicillin), insect bites or stings, or even intestinal parasites. The origin of "non-allergic" hives is more obscure, and treatment is less effective.

Treatment

Since hives are usually related to an allergic reaction, self-help therapy aims to discover the cause. This takes some detective work and, like a good gumshoe, you should keep a notebook. Record everything put into the mouth, including food, drink, drugs, and so forth—plus the onset of each crop of hives. Soon a pattern may emerge. Common culprits are chocolate, nuts, berries (especially the strawberry), seafood, pork, milk, and eggs. If hives seem to follow eating a certain food, eliminate it from the diet for two weeks, and see if the hives subside. If so, that food, let's say eggs, should be eliminated from the diet for six months, including all other foods (such as cake, pastry, noodles) that may also contain small amounts of the causative food. Sometimes, after the cause has been absent from the diet for six months, it is possible to ingest small amounts, although the hives victim should probably never again eat large quantities of any food that has been shown to produce hives. (A handy elimination diet is found under Food Allergies on page 120).

Hives following injections such as penicillin are a warning that subsequent use of the drug, even by mouth, but especially by injection, may be followed by a severe reaction. If a bee or wasp sting is followed by hives that cover the body, the physician often will recommend that desensitization injections begin, and he may advise that antihistamine or cortisone tablets be kept at home for emergency use.

Acute hives almost always subside spontaneously, and no treatment may be needed. Individual welts may disappear if cold packs are applied, and a tepid (about room temperature) bath may be soothing. Mild hives are sometimes treated with cortisone tablets such as prednisone or antihistamine tablets such as chlorpheniramine (Chlor-Trimeton). If severe, the doctor may give an injection of cortisone or even epinephrine (Adrenalin).

Since anxiety is often a factor in chronic recurrent hives, the sufferer should avoid stressful situations such as personal confrontations, anxiety-provoking responsibilities, and emotionally charged committee meetings. Also helpful may be a mild antihistamine-sedative such as Compoz or even a three-week vacation away from the tensions of home and work.

HYDROCELE

Synonym: fluid in the scrotum

The hydrocele is a fluid-filled sac in the scrotum adjacent to the testis, and is found in males of all ages, from newborn babies to senior citizens. No pain is involved, and the hydrocele is noted only as a soft scrotal swelling that transmits the glow of a flashlight (in contrast to more solid tissue, which will not transmit light).

Treatment

Three options are open in dealing with a hydrocele—observation, surgery, or needle removal of the fluid:

- Observation is recommended for hydroceles found in infant males, since many will resolve spontaneously. The hydrocele is watched and measured during the first few months of life, but if it shows no sign of disappearance, surgery is considered.
- Surgery is advised for most persistent hydroceles, particularly when a period of observation reveals no change in the size. Hospitalization will be needed, but the results of surgery are usually good.
- Needle removal (aspiration) is a poor third choice, recommended only for elderly individuals who are poor surgical risks. Relief is temporary at best, even when a cortisone compound is injected following removal of the fluid, and infection is a threat. And within a few months the hydrocele has filled again with fluid.

HYPERACTIVITY

Synonyms: hyperactive child, hyperkinesis, minimal brain dysfunction

"Joseph, sit still and pay attention." That's what the hyperactive child hears from morning 'til night. He suffers from a short attention span, is easily distracted, and is said to suffer "minimal brain dysfunction." Thus he's a handful at home and a special problem for the teacher in school, who sends Joseph and his parents to the doctor for medication.

Traditional therapy has been stimulants, including dextroamphetamine (Dexedrine), methylphenidate (Ritalin), and the newer pemoline (Cylert). Stimulants, whose use in an overactive child seems paradoxical, work by increasing his concentration abilities and lenghtening his attention span.

A self-help trial of stimulant therapy can give a clue to the outcome of drug treatment in the suspected hyperactive youngster: give him a cup of coffee for breakfast and observe the effect of caffeine.

Adjunctive therapy includes special learning techniques and psychological counseling.

There is a 1975 book that describes an interesting theory. In his book *Why Your Child Is Hyperactive* (Random House, New York), Ben F. Feingold, M.D., tells of favorable behavior and personality changes in the hyperactive child by removing all synthetic food coloring and artificial flavoring from his diet. The therapy is self-help, safe, and free; if your child is hyperactive, it's worth a try.

HYPERTENSION

Synonyms: essential hpertension, high blood pressure

More than 20 million Americans suffer hypertension, making high blood pressure one of the most widespread ailments discussed in this book. And hypertension is also one of the most important, since untreated or even inadequately treated high blood pressure can lead to heart attacks, strokes, and early death.

Early high blood pressure usually causes no symptoms, and the first knowledge of its presence may begin on a routine physical examination. The physician fits the blood pressure cuff (properly called a sphygmomanometer) around the arm. He inflates the bag within the cuff until arterial blood flow to the arm is blocked. Then the cuff pressure is gradually released as the physician listens at the elbow with his stethoscope. When the patient's arterial blood pressure first exceeds the pressure of the cuff, the doctor hears a rhythmic thump-thump-thump of the pulse beat. This upper level of blood pressure is called the systolic pressure and measures the force of the heartbeat. The physician continues to decrease the pressure within the cuff until the thump-thump-thump ceases; this level is the diastolic pressure, marking the resting pressure within the arteries.

What is normal? There's no easy answer to that question. What's acceptable for a 60-year-old would be hypertensive in a teenager. The average blood pressure increases with age, giving rise to the now-discredited formula that blood pressure equals one hundred plus your age. Rough normal figures are these: Teenagers will have blood pressure readings around 110/70, perhaps less, while healthy young adults will have blood pressures in the 120/80 range. During middle age, mean blood pressure readings rise to about 130/85, and middle-aged men with diastolic blood pressures of 90 to 99 have a mortality risk twice that of their normal counterparts. A blood pressure in excess of 150/100 is abnormal at any age.

The Origins of Hypertension

The doctor cheers when he finds a curable cause of one's blood pressure—a tumor (pheochromocytoma) of the adrenal gland or narrowing of the large artery to the kidney. But such causes are uncommon, and more than 95 percent of individuals with high blood pressure have "essential hypertension"—meaning that the exact cause is unknown.

While exact causes remain elusive, we know what contributes to high blood pressure. Racial ancestry plays a role; for example, hypertension among American blacks at middle age is at least twice that of whites. Family history is significant, and parents with high blood pressure beget offspring with an increased risk of early hypertension.

Each extra pound of body weight adds up to one mile of capillaries that the heart must pump blood through. Also increasing the heart's work (and thus the blood pressure) is the increased blood volume that follows high salt consumption, as salt draws fluid into the bloodstream.

Emotional stress adds to the high incidence of hypertension in this country, as Americans in all levels of society strive to cope with increased job pressures, domestic strife, rising prices, and oppressive taxes, not to mention impure air, noise pollution, and vanishing personal privacy.

Treating Hypertension

When the patient and physician work hand in hand, hypertension can almost always be controlled. It is important to realize that high blood pressure, once it has been diagnosed with certainty, is a lifelong affliction requiring continued treatment. The sphygmomanometer reading may return to normal once therapy is begun, but if treatment is stopped the blood pressure begins to rise.

Weight must be controlled. If you are above your ideal weight, and have gained more than a few pounds since age 25, blood pressure levels can be lowered as pounds melt away. In my office, I have been impressed by how a weight gain of five to ten pounds will be followed by a predictable rise in blood pressure of 8 to 10 points. And shedding the excess pounds is followed by a fall in the blood pressure. If you are overweight, self-help treatment begins with dietary control.

Salt contributes to high blood pressure, and self-help treatment includes salt restriction. Usually it's unnecessary to buy expensive salt-free foods, and blood pressure levels usually respond to elimination of inherently high-salt foods (such as ham, bacon, salted potato chips, and so forth) as well as banishing the salt shaker from the kitchen and dining room. By not adding salt in cooking or at the table, a significant degree of salt restriction is achieved.

Many hypertensives require both calorie and salt restriction; the following is a low-salt, calorie-controlled diet.

Low Salt, Low Calorie Diet

Foods Permitted	Foods to Be Avoided
Cereals	
Cooked oat and wheat cereals	Dry precooked cereals
Shredded wheat	Sugar-coated cereals
Wheatena	
Farina	
Bran cereals	
Breads	
Whole wheat bread	White bread
	Muffins, rolls, and biscuits
	Corn bread
	Pancakes and waffles
Soups	
Fresh soup with vegetables listed below	Creamed soups
	Meat stock soups
	Bean, lentil, or split pea soups
	Bouillon and broth

Foods Permitted	Foods to Be Avoided

Meat, Fish, and Dairy Products

Boiled, baked, or broiled veal, ham, lean beef turkey or chicken, and fish	Mutton and pork Fried or fatty meats Shellfish
Soft cooked eggs	Fried eggs
Cottage cheese	Cheese except cottage cheese

Vegetables

Cucumbers	Sweetened or canned vegetables
Carrots	Beets
Brussels sprouts	Peas
Onions	Potatoes
Lettuce	Spinach
Tomatoes	Corn
Cabbage	Celery
Broccoli	
Asparagus	
Green beans	
Squash	

Fruits

Pureed fruits	Sweetened or canned fruits
Fruit juices	Bananas
Apples	Dates
Apricots	Figs
Pears	Raisins
Prunes	
Oranges	
Pineapple	
Grapefruit	
Melons	
Plums	
Peaches	

Desserts

Fresh fruit	Pies and pastries
Gelatin	Custard and pudding
Cakes	Ice cream
	Sherbet
	Bread pudding
	Tapioca pudding
	Corn starch or rice pudding

Beverages

Coffee and tea	Alcohol
Decaffeinated coffee	Milk
Diet soda	

Foods Permitted	Foods to Be Avoided
Cocoa, Postum, and Ovaltine	
Skimmed milk	

Miscellaneous

Foods Permitted	Foods to Be Avoided
Liquid vegetable oils (corn, soybean, and safflower)	Animal fats and lard
Pepper	Sugar
Garlic	Salt
	Olives
	Nuts
	Pickles
	Macaroni and spaghetti
	Tomato paste
	Mayonnaise
	Gravy
	Mustard
	Horseradish
	Salted nuts
	Unsalted nuts
	Jelly and jam
	Relish
	Vinegar
	Candy

Smoking can raise the diastolic blood pressure and should be avoided by all hypertensive individuals.

Minimize anxiety, sidestepping situations that build up tension day by day. Avoid irritating individuals and exasperating confrontations, while cultivating the equanimity that helps subdue a bounding blood pressure. A good natural sedative is camomile with honey.

Drug therapy of hypertension offers the physician a wide range of therapeutic choices, and medicines are often used in a pyramidal fashion, with each therapeutic step building upon the last, as illustrated in Figure 16. Medicines prescribed to treat high blood pressure may include:

- Diuretics, which remove excess salt and fluid from the bloodstream and are the first-choice drugs of most physicians treating high blood pressure. Many brands are available, and favorites include chlorothiazide (Diuril), hydrochlorothiazide (Esidrix), furoxemide (Lasix), chlorthalidone (Hygroton), and others. Ex-

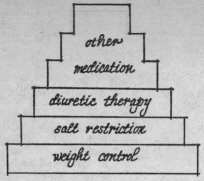

FIGURE 16. *Steps in the treatment of hypertension.*

cessive potassium loss may be a problem, manifested as weakness and possible heart irregularities if the patient is taking digitalis; potassium replacement with orange juice, bananas, or potassium supplements avoids this complication.

- Reserpine and its derivatives, which lower blood pressure at the risk of lethargy, nasal stuffiness, and depression.
- Hydralazine (Apresoline), a more potent blood pressure depressant although its use may strain an already weakened heart.
- Guanethidine (Ismelin), which lowers blood pressure by blocking nerve transmission to the walls of arteries. It lowers blood pressure efficiently, at the risk of lightheadedness upon standing abruptly.
- Methyldopa (Aldomet), which combats blood pressure-raising chemical compounds, and is particularly useful in hypertensive individuals who suffer kidney disease. The need for two to four daily doses makes methyldopa les convenient than other once-a-day medications.
- Clonidine (Catapres), which requires only two daily doses to lower blood pressure; side effects include sedation and dry mouth.
- Propranolol (Inderal), which can slow the heart rate and prevent angina pectoris as well as control hyper-

172

tension. Often used in tandem with Apresoline (hydralazine), propranolol may aggravate asthma, diabetes, and congestive heart failure.
- Emergency antihypertensive drugs, used when soaring blood pressure levels bring the threat of stroke, such as diazoxide (Hyperstat) and sodium nitroprusside.

The control of high blood pressure can add years to your life, and life insurance companies have accurately documented the risk of even mild hypertension. If your blood pressure is above normal, even if only a few points, follow the self-help suggestions listed here and see your doctor for regular checkups. Controlling high blood pressure may not make you feel better (since modest blood pressure elevations cause no symptoms), but hypertension therapy pays dividends of longer life, uncomplicated by the cardiovascular consequences of poorly controlled hypertension.

For further information about hypertension write to:

The American Heart Association, Inc.
7320 Greenville Avenue
Dallas, Texas 75231

National High Blood Pressure Education Program
National Heart and Lung Institute
Washington, D.C. 20015

HYPOGLYCEMIA

Synonyms: low blood sugar, functional hypoglycemia

Although low blood sugar reactions may occur following the administration of insulin, functional hypoglycemia describes the spontaneous incidence of low blood sugar levels when no insulin or other medication has been given. The victim notes a weak, faint jittery feeling associated with sweating. The reaction usually begins several hours after a meal, and is promptly relieved by orange juice, candy, or other high-sugar food.

Functional hypoglycemia causes bouncing blood sugar levels. When carbohydrates are eaten, the blood sugar level rises quickly, often to heights consistent with diabetes (and in fact, victims of functional hypoglycemia often develop diabetes in

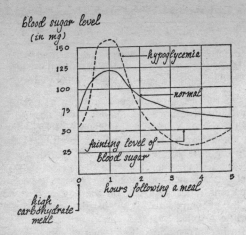

FIGURE 17. *Blood sugar levels in hypoglycemia.*

later life). Then the blood sugar plunges to a low level, usually below 50 mg per 100 cc and symptoms begin (see Figure 17). Since, of all body tissues, the brain is most dependent upon blood sugar levels, mental symptoms such as anxiousness and impaired concentration may occur first. The diagnosis is suspected from one's medical history and confirmed by a five-hour glucose tolerance test.

Avoiding Hypoglycemia

Functional hypoglycemia is treated by diet alone. Since the cause is a cockeyed metabolism of sugars, the treatment is a diet low in sugar and high in protein, with six small feedings taken daily to avoid peaks and valleys in blood sugar levels. The following diet will control most functional hypoglycemia.

General Diet Rules
1. Take six small meals daily, with protein such as meat, fish, cheese, or egg in each meal.
2. Avoid alcohol.
3. Don't smoke.
4. Take a multivitamin such as Optilet-M-500 once daily.
5. Be careful of portion sizes; don't overeat and gain weight.

Low Carbohydrate, High Protein Hypoglycemia Diet

Foods Permitted	*Foods to Be Avoided*

Cereals

Cooked oats and cereals	Dry precooked cereals
Bran cereals	Sugar-coated cereals

Breads

Whole wheat bread	White bread
Corn bread	Muffins, rolls, and biscuits
	Pancakes and waffles

Soups

Creamed soups
Meat stock soups
Bean, lentil, or split pea soups
Bouillon and broth

Meat, Fish, and Dairy Products

Boiled, baked, or broiled	Fried or fatty meats
veal, ham, lean beef	Fried eggs
turkey or chicken, and fish	
Mutton and pork	
Shellfish	
Soft cooked eggs	
Cheese	
Cottage cheese	

Vegetables

All raw, cooked, or pureed unsweetened vegetables	Vegetables that have been candied, sweetened, or packed in syrup

Fruits

All raw, cooked, or pureed unsweetened fruits,	Fruits that have been candied, sweetened, or packed in syrup

Desserts

Fresh fruit	Cake
Gelatin	Pies and pastries
Junket	Custard and pudding
	Ice cream
	Sherbet
	Bread, rice, or tapioca puddings

Foods Permitted	Foods to Be Avoided
Beverages	
Fat-free milk	Coffee
Weak tea	Alcohol
Decaffeinated coffee	Cocoa, Postum, and Ovaltine
Diet soda	Whole milk
Miscellaneous	
Liquid vegetable oils (corn, soybean, and safflower)	Animal fats and lard
	Sugar
Salt	Olives
Pepper	Macaroni and spaghetti
Pickles	Garlic
Tomato paste	Mayonnaise
Mustard	Gravy
Horseradish	Salted nuts
Relish	Unsalted nuts
Vinegar	Jelly and jam
	Candy
	Honey and molasses

IMMUNIZATIONS

The civilized world is relatively free of smallpox, tetanus, polio, and a number of other infectious diseases—not because we have discovered cures for these maladies (which we haven't), but because medical science has developed first-rate vaccines that can prevent them.

Their worth well established by scientific studies and decades of use, routine immunizations should begin in infants at two months of age, with booster doses of certain vaccines continued throughout life.

The following immunization schedule has been approved by the American Academy of Family Physicians.

Recommended Immunization Schedule:
Your Personal Checklist

Age	Immunization	Date Received
2 months	DPT No. 1 (Diphtheria-Pertussis-Tetanus)	_____
	Sabin Trivalent Oral Polio No. 1	_____

176

Age	Immunization	Date Received
4 months	DPT No. 2	_____
	Sabin Trivalent Oral Polio No. 2	_____
6 months	DPT No. 3	_____
	Sabin Trivalent Oral Polio No. 3	_____
9 months	Tine Tuberculosis Skin Test	_____
15 months	Live Measles Vaccine	_____
	Live Mumps Vaccine	_____
	Live Rubella (German Measles) Vaccine	_____
	Smallpox Vaccination (given following the first birthday if recommended by the physician. The United States Public Health Service states that routine smallpox vaccination is not needed, but some experts disagree.)	_____
18 months	DPT Booster	_____
	Sabin Trivalent Oral Polio Booster	_____
5 years	DPT Booster	_____
	Sabin Trivalent Oral Polio Booster	_____
Remainder of Life	Adult Type Td (Tetanus-Diphtheria) Booster every ten years	_____
	No tetanus booster is needed for clean minor wounds unless more than ten years have elapsed since the last dose of tetanus toxoid. If a contaminated tetanus-prone wound is sustained, a booster dose should be given if more than five years have passed since the last dose of tetanus toxoid.	_____

IMPETIGO

Synonym: impetigo contagiosa
Impetigo is a bacterial infection of the skin, often found in

young children during summer months when germs find a safe haven in tiny scratches caked with sweat and dirt. Once on fertile ground, the staphyloccus or streptococcus bacteria begin to multiply, causing a crusted infection that may spread to nearby areas and to others in the household. Impetigo often involves the face and may complicate a nasal discharge to cold sore of the lip.

Although usually a not-to-serious infection, streptococcal impetigo occasionally leads to formidable aftereffects, including rheumatic fever or glomerulonephritis (*q.v.*).

Attacking Impetigo

Since it's always preferable to prevent rather than treat disease, mothers should insist that their children take (as, indeed, all individuals should) a daily thorough bath or shower. All tiny cuts and scratches should be treated promptly with soap-and-water scrubbing, followed by a disinfectant such as povidone-iodine (Betadine).

Tiny patches of impetigo are often amenable to home care. Scrub vigorously with soap and water, being careful to remove the scabs beneath which bacteria lurk. Dry carefully, then apply nonprescription Bacitracin Ointment and leave open to the air. Most minor impetigo infections will subside within a few days.

If the skin infection fails to respond promptly or if it is widespread, see the doctor. In addition to scrubbing and the application of an antibiotic ointment, he will often prescribe an antibiotic to be taken by mouth, such as penicillin or erythromycin (Ilosone or Erythrocin), giving stubborn impetigo the knockout punch.

IMPOTENCE

Synonym: male sexual dysfunction

Impotence is the failure of the male to achieve and maintain a satisfactory erection during the sex act. Mercifully, most cases are transitory—related to anxiety, guilt, and undue haste. The technical term is "performance anxiety," the fear of failure. One or two unsuccessful attempts serve to erode the male's confidence, and subsequent sex acts are seen as a physical challenge rather than a pleasurable experience. The anxious male enters the bedroom thinking, "I failed last time and the time before, and I'll probably fail again now."

Overcoming Impotence

A few diseases may possibly cause impotence—diabetes, alcoholism, disorders of the nerves, a blood clot in the aorta (Leriché syndrome), and other less likely ailments. These disorders are rarely the origin of impotence, however, and treatment usually involves one or more of the measures described next.

Since anxiety plays a major role, the doctor may prescribe a mild tranquilizer such as chlordiazepoxide (Librium) to be taken several times daily, or perhaps in anticipation of a sexual encounter. Or the prescription may be merely a quiet drink with the sexual partner before bedtime.

Sometimes prescribed are male hormones, vitamins, and/or thyroid extract; one such combination is Android Tablets, taken one to three times daily. Naturalists tell us that sexual potency is enhanced by eating certain foods, including celery, pineapple, and oats. (Could this be the origin of "sowing wild oats"?) The benefits of such therapy are disputed, and their effect may be more psychological than physical.

Boredom often plays a role, with mechanical embraces and predictable positions eliminating the excitement of the sex act. I sometimes advise couples to read *The Joy of Sex* together, and I encourage them to explore new techniques. A vacation often helps, even a weekend at a nearby motel.

When impotence occurs, it's a problem for both him and her. His mate's support should be elicited in stimulating an erection, aiding entry even when tumescence is less than complete, and bolstering the male's lagging confidence.

Sex clinics à la Masters and Johnson are now in vogue. These help patients explore their sexuality, teach helpful techniques, and aid in building lost confidence. A favorite ploy is touching—experiencing tactile sensitivity with attempted intercourse forbidden, heightening interpersonal feelings and enhancing sexuality while removing the threat of failure. Ethical clinics perform a valued service for their patients, but before undertaking such therapy, you and your doctor should carefully check the credentials of the therapist. (Pioneer sex therapist William H. Masters has charged that up to 99 percent of sex clinics "are run by charlatans for money.")

Almost all impotence can be overcome, and much of the treatment is of self-help nature, with information guided by professional counseling.

For further information about sexuality write to:

American Association of Sex Educators, Counselors, and Therapists
Suite 304
5010 Wisconsin Ave., N.W.
Washington, D.C. 20016

Sex Information and Education Council of the U.S.
137 North Franklin Street
Hempstead, New York 11550

INFECTIOUS MONONUCLEOSIS

Synonyms: infectious "mono," the kissing disease, "mono"
Infectious mononucleosis is a disease of young persons, and received its nickname "the kissing disease" when Colonel Robert J. Hoagland, Chief of the Army Hospital at West Point, linked its occurrence in cadets to their weekend osculatory adventures with visiting coeds. Lassitude is the universal symptom and most patients suffer sore throat and enlarged lymph glands of the neck. A low-grade fever is usually found, and there may be a skin rash, plus enlargement of the liver and/or spleen. The cause appears to be a microorganism called the Epstein-Barr virus, also implicated in certain lymphomas.

The doctor clinches the diagnosis with a blood count. No specific cure is available, but infectious mononucleosis usually subsides spontaneously within three to six weeks.

Treatment

Rest is the cornerstone of therapy, with school attendance usually prohibited until acute symptoms subside, and strenuous physical exertion avoided until the patient is pronounced thoroughly cured. Contact sports are prohibited since trauma could cause rupture of an enlarged spleen.

Vitamins such as Theragran or Daylet-M are often advised, and aspirin is taken as needed for fever. If a strep throat infection is present, the physician may prescribe penicillin or erythromycin (Ilosone), and cortisone is sometimes given in severe cases. Avoid the use of ampicillin, since use of this antibiotic is very likely to cause a rash in the patient with "mono."

Upon recovery, a gradual return to activity is advised. Keep a wary eye out for recurrent symptoms of lassitude, fever, and sore throat.

INFLUENZA

Synonyms: viral influenza, flu, Asian flu, grippe

This is another ailment for which you can (and usually should) save the expense and hassle of an office call. Unless the patient suffers one of the bacterial complications mentioned below, he should be kept in bed and out of the doctor's waiting room.

The flu begins with chills and fever, plus overwhelming fatigue. Headache is often a prominent symptom, there will be a loss of appetite, and the patient describes himself as too weak to roll over in bed. Associated symptoms of less severity may include slight sore throat, minimal cough, and scant abdominal cramps.

Treatment

Mother always recommended treating the flu with bed rest, fluids, and aspirin. Mother was right!

Rarely need the flu victim be advised to take to bed; he's there already. The lethargy that accompanies flu is overwhelming, especially when capped by fever up to 105 degrees. Bed rest is enforced until acute symptoms have subsided, and the flu victim should spend a few extra days resting at home, lest a premature return to work be followed by recurrence of symptoms.

Aspirin, or perhaps acetaminophen (Tylenol), is still the mainstay of flu therapy. Two aspirin or Tylenol tablets are administered every six hours when fever and achiness are present—but should be omitted if symptoms are minimal;

there's nothing to be gained by administering aspirin to alleviate symptoms that have subsided, and aspirin overdosage may cause stomach irritation and ringing in the ears. Propoxyphene (Darvon) and similar strong analgesics lack aspirin's fever-fighting potency and offer no advantage.

Naturalists believe that early flu symptoms sometimes respond to large doses of lecithin. At the first hint of achiness or fever, take one tablespoonful of liquid lecithin—a phospholipid available at health food stores. Continue to take one tablespoonfull of liquid lecithin or ten 1,200-mg lecithin capsules every eight hours for two days to abort the early symptoms of a viral flu.

Fluids are all the nourishment the flu victim feels up to taking, and he can do without solid foods for a few days. Suggested liquids that may prove palatable and will help prevent dehydration are:

Water at room temperature
Weak tea
Dilute fruit juice
Jello water
Cola syrup in water
Weak bouillon
Ginger ale

In addition to the above, patience is prescribed for the flu victim. Regardless of the treatment, he'll feel miserable for at least several days. One week away from work is about average, and he'll feel weak, with a tendency toward lightheadedness and easy sweating, for another 7 to 14 days.

What the Doctor Can Do about the Flu

There is some evidence that amantadine (Symmetrel) can abort some very early cases of flu if taken at the first sign of symptoms, although the original use of this medication was prophylaxis of influenza Type A_2, and the drug has also been prescribed to treat Parkinson's disease. But treatment of flu with amantadine lacks FDA approval and is therefore prescribed infrequently for this purpose.

Antibiotics are of no value in acute but uncomplicated viral influenza and there is some evidence to indicate that they may be harmful: when administered without good reason, penicillin or other antibiotics seem to assure that resistant germs will cause complications. Your doctor knows this, and don't try to talk him into "a shot of penicillin" for simple flu.

On the other hand, if the flu becomes complicated by an acute ear infection, bacterial throat infection, or perhaps even pneumonia, then antibiotics can be lifesaving.

Preventing Flu

Avoiding viral influenza should be a prime goal during the winter months. Begin with a dose of common sense: Take plenty of fruit juices for Vitamin C, get your share of rest, stay away from crowds, and particularly avoid individuals who have the flu.

Flu shots are strongly recommended for the elderly and for individuals with chronic diseases such as asthma or heart disease that might cause complications if the flu occurred. Some physicians suggest flu shots for all adults who would suffer financial loss and severe inconvenience if they contracted a week-long energy-draining illness; but that includes about all of us, doesn't it?

Flu shots may be administered the first cool day in autumn and should certainly be given by mid-November. The dose is one 0.5-cc shot annually, if you have no allergy to eggs, chicken, or feathers.

For more information on influenza write to:

National Communicable Disease Center
Atlanta, Georgia 30334

INGROWN TOENAIL

Four factors favor the ingrown toenail. There's often a family history of ingrown toenails, with the tendency for toenail troubles to pass from generation to generation. Tight-fitting shoes and stockings play a role, squeezing tender tissues against an unyielding nail. Ingrown toenails often accompany obesity, with flabby skin rising to engulf the nail painfully. And finally, the ingrown toenail often arises from improper nail-cutting, as toenails are rounded like fingernails, rather than cut straight across—the proper way to trim toenails (see Figure 18).

The ingrown toenail causes pain and swelling and seems to scream for attention.

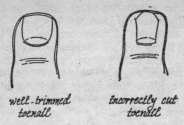

well-trimmed toenail   incorrectly cut toenail

FIGURE 18. *Properly and improperly trimmed toenails.*

Preventing and Treating the Ingrown Toenail

To avoid ingrown toenails, treat the factors over which you have control. Your family tree can't be altered, but excess pounds can be shed and footwear should be selected so that shoes and socks don't pinch the toes. Careful trimming of the nails to allow square corners prevents rounded edges from digging into adjacent tissues.

A mild ingrown toenail can often be treated, or even prevented, by tucking a small wad of cotton under the nail's corner, covered by flexible collodion (no prescription needed) or even a light coating of Duco Household Cement. When properly "glued," the wad of cotton will remain in place for several weeks, even surviving showering, and will guide the nail's growth out of the adjacent skin and into proper alignment.

Infected or severely ingrown nails sometimes require surgery, and this is a job for the physician. Often he will remove a quarter-inch margin of nail, perhaps along with a wedge of adjacent skin, and following surgery may recommend warm saline soaks thrice daily until all inflammation subsides.

INSECT STINGS

Synonyms: bee, wasp, hornet, or yellow-jacket stings
The sting on any of the hymenoptera family of insects not

only hurts like blazes, it can threaten the life of allergic individuals. Many cases of sudden death occurring outdoors are attributed to heart attacks or strokes, yet are in reality sudden overwhelming allergic reactions to insect stings. Not confined to adults, severe allergic episodes following hymenoptera stings are not uncommon in youngsters.

Often insect stings can be prevented. Bees and their cousins are attracted to bright colored clothing, as well as to scents of perfume, lipstick, and other cosmetic products; the bee hovers hopefully as though you were a gay sweet-smelling flower. When working outdoors, there's less chance of being stung if you bathe with an odorless soap, wear not-too-bright clothing, and shun aromatic cosmetics.

If a curious bee comes by, stand quietly. He may buzz and investigate but won't attack unless startled by a quick movement. Even a bee walking on your arm or leg is unlikely to sting unless in self-defense.

Treating the Insect Sting

If stung, apply ice as soon as possible, reducing blood flow to the area. Sit quietly to reduce circulation and minimize the spread of venom throughout the body. If there is no history or suspicion of allergy, this is all the self-help therapy needed. Realize that an insect sting will be swollen and painful for several days, with prodigious swelling if the sting occurs near the easily stretched tissues of the back of the hands or around the eyes. Ice helps reduce the swelling, aspirin alleviates discomfort, and time heals the sting.

Meat tenderizer can help reduce pain and swelling after a sting. Sprinkle ordinary grocery-store meat tenderizer on a moist gauze pad, and hold tightly against the sting for one hour. Dr. Roy Kulland of North Dakota writes in *Continuing Education*, July 1974, "It is amazing at the end of twenty minutes to one-half hour how much it had reduced the swelling and the pain was practically gone shortly after applying the meat tenderizer."

It's a different story when allergy is present. The individual allergic to hymenoptera stings may develop only an itching skin rash. But more dangerous is swelling of the windpipe, which impairs breathing, and falling blood pressure, which can cause shock. If stung, the allergic individual should start for the nearest medical facility without waiting to see if a reaction occurs. If handy along the way, it's helpful to apply ice. A tourniquet such as a rolled handkerchief knotted above the sting helps impede absorption.

If there is a known history of allergy to stinging insects, it's prudent to have on hand medication to take when stung. Some physicians prefer the use of an antihistamine such as diphenhydramine (Benadryl); others instruct their patients to take two to four prednisone tablets if stung. No prescription is needed for Primatene Aerosol Mist containing epinephrine— potentially lifesaving when swelling blocks air passages. Or the doctor may recommend a more potent inhaler such as Medihaler-Epi, containing a larger dose of epinephrine per inhalation. Sometimes used is a special emergency insect-sting treatment kit called ANA-KIT, available from Hollister-Stier Laboratories, 3525 North Regal Street, Box 3145, Terminal Annex, Spokane, Washington 99220.

INSOMNIA

Synonym: sleeplessness

For one reason or another, sleeplessness comes to all of us sooner or later. There is almost always a cause, and when it is found, the cure is usually painfully obvious:

- Stimulants, particularly coffee containing caffeine, can disturb restful sleep. Switch to Sanka or Brim—or eliminate coffee altogether—and restful sleep often follows.
- Afternoon naps can interfere with nocturnal slumber. If bedtime insomnia follows an after-lunch snooze, resolve now to stay awake until ready to retire for the night.
- Excitement, or even arguments at bedtime, can delay restful sleep. Prepare for slumber by beginning to relax a few hours before retiring. Watch a soporific television comedy, then read in bed before turning off the light. Don't try to be clever or creative just before bedtime or your mind will keep churning after lights out.
- Bedtime snacks delay slumber in some individuals, and encourage sleep in others. If you are having trou-

ble falling asleep at night, examine your evening eating habits.

- A too-hot or too-cold room interferes with restful sleep, often manifested as awakening with a chill or with overdried respiratory passages. Problems arise when hothouse Mary marries outdoor Jim who likes the windows wide open, but they must seek a common ground if both are to enjoy a good night's sleep.
- An uncomfortable mattress is a common cause of sleeplessness. You spend one-third of your life in bed; pay the price for a top-quality mattress and spring, and be sure that the firmness is right for you.
- Insomnia can accompany physical disorders, such as nocturnal leg cramps, asthma, congestive heart failure, peptic ulcer, chronic diarrhea, and more. Treat the disease and restful sleep will follow.

What about Sedatives?

Bedtime sedatives are not the easy answer to insomnia. In fact they're not an answer at all but should be viewed as a temporary crutch until healthful sleep patterns have been formed. If you plan to take a sedative at bedtime, understand the drug you are taking, including its limitations and hazards.

A favorite folk-medicine sedative is common lettuce (Lactuca sativa and Luctuca virosa), its calming properties attributed to lactucarium. Possible uses include raw leaves, lettuce syrup or alcohol solution, lettuce leaf broth, pills, or lettuce seed tea. The sedative properties of lettuce, plus the natural medical uses of most common vegetables and fruits, are described in *Organic Garden Medicine*, by Jean Valnet, M.D. (Erbonia Books, New Paltz, New York).

Available over-the-counter are a number of sleep-inducers. Most contain pyrilamine and methapyrilene—antihistamines that cause drowsiness. Some also contain scopolamine, a derivative of belladonna. Good choices include:

- Nytol Capsules, containing 50 mg of methapyrilene.
- Sleep-Eze Tablets containing 25 mg methapyrilene and 0.125 mg scopolamine.
- Sominex Tablets containing 0.25 mg scopolamine, 25 mg methapyrilene, and 200 mg salicylamide.

Stronger sedatives require a prescription and carry a risk of habituation. If symptoms warrant their use, the doctor may prescribe one of the following sedatives:

- Chloral hydrate (Noctec) is a time-honored, reliable, safe sleeping capsule.
- Ethchlorvynol (Placidyl) usually induces sleep promptly and is less potent than the barbiturates.
- Glutethimide (Doriden) is an effective sedative that some doctors consider to have a lesser margin of safety than the barbiturates. The addiction risk is fairly high.
- Fluorazepam (Dalmane) is a sedative that seems effective and safe.
- Pentobarbital (Nembutal), one of the several barbiturates available by prescription, is a potent sedative sometimes recommended for stubborn insomnia.

There are many more sleeping pills that I could name. They all share characteristics with one or more of the above and all are potentially habit-forming. The definitive treatment of insomnia should be self-help—the elimination of the cause of sleeplessnes, leading to restful drug-free slumber.

If you would like to learn more about sleep, read *Sleep: The Gentle Tyrant* by Wilse B. Webb (Prentice-Hall, Englewood Cliffs, New Jersey), discussing body rhythms, changes in sleep patterns with age, and sleep disorders.

JOCK ITCH

Synonyms: groin itch, crotch itch, intertrigo of the groin

So called because it strikes the area where a "jock strap" is worn, jock itch commonly afflicts athletes, although inflammation of the groin and perineal area can occur in individuals of all ages and sexes, regardless of their athletic activities.

Jock itch begins as chafing, with perspiration, warmth, and rubbing of opposing tissues causing skin irritation. Redness and inflammation occur, often abetted by scratching. Next may come infection with bacteria, fungi, or yeast organisms (Candida).

Get the jump on jock itch by applications of powder to prevent unncessary wetness and chafing. Good products include:

- Cruex Spray-on Powder containing one percent hexachlorophene and 10 percent calcium undecylenate in a talc base.
- Sopronol Powder containing sodium caprylate and propionate plus zinc propionate.
- Johnson's Baby Powder containing talc.

Infections of this area are common. Frequent invaders are yeast and fungus germs, both often responding to applications of Lotrimin brand of clortrimazole cream (prescription needed) three times daily.

Over-the-counter tolnaftate (Tinactin) cream and solution work well against fungus infections, but won't cure Candida; neither clortrimazole nor tolnaftate is effective against bacteria.

Bacterial infections respond best to warm salt water soaks for one-half hour three times daily, followed by the local application of Bacitracin Ointment, perhaps supplemented by an oral antibiotic prescribed by the doctor. For more detailed discussion of fungus, Candida, and bacterial skin infections, see Candidiasis, Fungus Infections, and Impetigo.

Other helpful measures include washing undergarments with a mild detergent, avoiding nylon or other synthetic underwear, and affording the "jock" area the best ventilation possible.

KERATOSIS

Synonyms: solar keratosis, farmer's skin, sailor's skin

The brown, dry, elevated patch seen on aging skin is called a keratosis. It forms on areas that have received repeated summer tans, and persons whose skin is weathered by many years of life outdoors may have dozens of keratoses. Usually, the keratosis is a harmless cosmetic nuisance, but occasionally one masks a skin cancer with malignant change signaled by crusting and bleeding.

Treatment

Keratoses usually afflict elderly individuals who have the good sense to leave them alone. However, some are rubbed by a collar or bra, while still others are considered cosmetically intolerable by the patient; these should be removed surgically. Following the injection of a local anesthetic, the keratosis is lightly desiccated (dried) with an electric needle, then scraped away.

Castor oil will sometimes remove a keratosis if applied once or twice daily for several months or more. If relief is not obtained, show the keratosis to the doctor.

Widespread keratoses—too many for simple surgical removal—can be treated with fluorouracil (Efudex) cream. Efudex is applied twice daily using a glove or nonmetal applicator. First comes redness, then blisters, then an ulceration, followed by healing with normal skin. The course of treatment lasts two to four weeks, should be undertaken only under medical supervision, and is not for the faint of heart.

KIDNEY STONE

Synonyms: urolithiasis, renal colic

The kidney stone causes no problem until it begins migration from the kidney to the bladder via the ureter (see Figure 19). Then the stone, usually little larger than a pinhead, causes excruciating discomfort as it is slowly pushed down the ureter by pressure from the kidney above. The pain of the kidney stone is said to equal the pain of childbirth (so said by doctors who have usually experienced neither).

The pain caused by a moving stone, called renal colic, comes and goes. It may seem to subside altogether, then recur as pressure builds again behind the stone. Eventually, most stones reach the bladder, and pain ceases abruptly. With the next act of urination, the stone is eliminated.

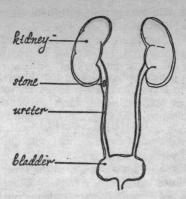

FIGURE 19. *Stone migrating from right kidney to bladder.*

Helping the Kidney Stone Along

The treatment of a kidney stone requires medical supervision, not only for the relief of pain, but to plan for the possibility that the stone may not pass spontaneously. The doctor may try to extract a stone that does not move with instruments inserted via the bladder, although an occasional stone must be removed surgically to prevent further damage to the kidney.

In the meantime, the patient who is passing a kidney stone can aid its progress:

- Stay active. Resting in bed will slow the movement of the stone, while walking about encourages its forward passage.
- Drink lots of fluids, to help flush the stone down the ureter and out of the urinary tract.
- Strain the urine through muslin or a linen handkerchief to catch the stone when passed. Stone analysis is a useful guide to future therapy.

Once the stone has passed, you and the doctor must consider possible causes. Has there been too much dietary calcium (taken as the treatment of gastritis or a peptic ulcer, perhaps)? Occasionally urinary stones follow overuse of Vitamin D. Uric acid stones are common in gout patients, particularly if they have taken medicine such as probenecid to increase the urinary flow of uric acid and have failed to follow the doctor's advice to drink two quarts of water daily. Whatever the cause, future stones are best prevented by taking plenty of fluids to retard crystal formation in the urine, and following the doctor's directions and diet to the letter.

LABYRINTHITIS

Synonyms: vertigo, dizziness

Labyrinthitis is an inflammation of the inner ear that disturbs the delicate balance mechanism. Victims complain of vertigo—dizziness described as whirling—usually beginning abruptly when the head is turned or upon standing quickly. Symptoms may be severe, and often interfere with walking or driving.

Labyrinthitis is usually caused by a viral infection, and subsides spontaneously after a few weeks, although some victims complain of transient episodes of vertigo that last for several months. Less common causes of labyrinthitis include drug toxicity (including salicylates, quinine, and certain antibiotics), bacterial infections, Meniere's disease (*q.v.*), and tumors.

What to Do about Labyrinthitis

See the doctor. It's important that the blood pressure be checked and that the physician exclude causes other than a simple viral infection.

Often useful are nonprescription pills to reduce vertigo, such as meclizine (Bonine) in 25-mg chewable tablets taken every 12 to 24 hours to relieve symptoms.

General measures to prevent episodes of vertigo include:

- Move the head slowly. Don't roll rapidly in bed or turn quickly to look behind you, since such rapid head movement is often followed by acute vertigo.
- Arise slowly from a sitting position. Standing abruptly often causes symptoms.
- Don't take aspirin or other products that might aggravate inner ear disorders.

- Get plenty of rest to speed recovery from viral labyrinthitis.
- Don't operate machinery (including an automobile) as a sudden episode of dizziness might jeopardize your safety.

LACERATION

Synonym: cut in the skin

A kitchen knife, piece of broken glass, or fall against a coffee table may cut the skin, and the extent of the injury may vary from a tiny puncture wound after stepping on a nail to a deep gash several inches long. Some lacerations are amenable to self-help therapy, while others demand skilled medical attention. In dealing with a laceration, the extent of bleeding, possible contamination that could lead to infection, the appearance of the wound, and tetanus prophylaxis must be considered.

Treatment

Virtually all lacerations bleed, and a tiny artery is sometimes severed, causing a pumping blood flow. Most likely to bleed profusely are cuts about the head, face, and neck—all areas of abundant blood supply. Bleeding can usually be controlled by firm pressure applied using a clean gauze compress—or, in an emergencey, a clean handkerchief or other absorbent material. Maintain pressure for several minutes, allowing time for blood clotting; resist the urge to peek every few seconds. Once the acute blood flow has stopped, further wound therapy can be undertaken.

Lacerations should be thoroughly cleaned. The doctor will often use Zephiran; Bactine is fine; but ordinary soap and water remain first-rate wound cleansers. Cleanse a wide margin—two or three inches—about the wound, and use copious quantities of water to flush away bacteria and debris. Following careful cleansing, an antiseptic solution is applied; a good choice is povidone-iodine (Betadine).

With bleeding stopped and the wound carefully cleansed, it's time to consider repair of the laceration. Patients with deep lacerations exposing underlying tissues, cuts more than one inch long, or wounds that gape apart should be rushed to the doctor or hospital. All shallow lacerations (one-half inch long or less) or larger lacerations occurring while in remote areas (where there will be a delay in reaching medical care) can be closed with butterflies. The doctor will often butterfly wounds using Steristrips—a special adhesive tape used to close small lacerations and even surgical wounds. But a makeshift butterfly can be cut from any surgical adhesive tape or even Scotch Magic Mending Tape (see Figure 20). One or more butterflies are placed across the laceration, easing tension on the scab and preventing separation of the wound edges. Butterfly closures have the advantage of not causing stitch marks, but fail to approximate deep tissues as well as stitches could; if in doubt, have the wound examined by the doctor.

A good natural remedy for small lacerations is a poultice of raw grated potatoes, applied repeatedly to help prevent infection and aid healing. Applications of cabbage juice or boiled cabbage leaves seem to achieve the same purpose.

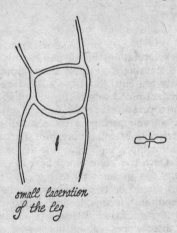

small laceration
of the leg

FIGURE 20. *Butterfly bandage to close a small cut.*

Tetanus occurs as germs enter the cut and grow within the tissues, producing a poisonous toxin. Careful cleansing of wounds helps expel possible tetanus-germ contamination, and tetanus prophylaxis must be considered whenever a laceration occurs. There is no hard-and-fast rule. Considered tetanus-prone are barnyard injuries (tetanus lives in the intestinal tracts of animals and is passed out with their droppings), extensive lacerations in which tetanus germs may be imbedded in torn tissues, or puncture wounds that may inject tetanus germs deep beneath the skin. Tetanus immunizations provide remarkably good protection if kept up to date. At present, doctors believe that a full tetanus series or tetanus series supplemented by booster shots provides solid protection for up to five years. Thus with a clean minor laceration, no tetanus booster should be needed if the last tetanus injection was given within five years, although the doctor may elect to update prophylaxis in cases of serious injury or doubtful tetanus immunization.

LEG CRAMPS

Leg cramps are a common complaint of older individuals. However, they may occur at any age as sudden tightening of the leg muscles awakens the sufferer from sleep and he bounds from the bed to stretch the leg and overcome the painful muscle tightness.

Sometimes the cause of leg cramps is apparent. Athletes may suffer muscle tightness following active exercise, and the weekend sportsman may experience nocturnal muscle cramps after a period of unaccustomed physical activity. Pregnancy sometimes causes leg cramps, as may diuretic therapy.

Treatment

Leg cramps due to physical exercise can be relieved by conditioning; daily physical exercise, including jogging, builds muscle tone and can help prevent leg cramps.

When leg cramps accompany pregnancy, diuretic therapy, or other conditions that change the body's metabolism, the doctor may prescribe a calcium lactate tablet to be taken three times daily, or perhaps an eight-ounce glass of orange juice each morning to combat potassium loss due to diuretics.

In most cases, the cause of leg cramps is obscure, and a time-honored treatment is a 300-mg quinine tablet taken at bedtime. Quinine breaks the rhythm of spasmodic muscular contractions, and the single bedtime dose usually is sufficient to prevent nocturnal leg cramps.

LICE

Synonyms: pediculosis, crabs

Surprising as it may seem, authorities estimate that more than two million Americans contract lice each year, and the incidence is increasing annually. Although once thought to be the special problem of the unwashed and underprivileged, lice today may be found on well-scrubbed middle-class people and their offspring.

Three distinct types of lice are found. The body louse, largest and longest of all, may occur anywhere on the body, and its bite may carry relapsing fever, trench fever, or typhus. The head louse is smaller, has long been the scourge of children's summer camps, and its favorite habitat is long unkempt hair, although is may migrate to the eyebrows or beard. The third member of the trio is the crab louse, whose numbers have increased with the rising incidence of venereal disease, since the crab louse may be spread through sexual intercourse as well as by contaminated bedding, clothing, or even toilet seats.

Lice soon make their presence known by tiny red bites associated with intense itching, and often followed by bacterial infection.

Licking the Louse Infestation

Medication will be needed, and the over-the-counter favorite is A-200 Pyrinate, a preparation of pyrethrins, piperonyl butoxide, and deodorized kerosene. A-200 Pyrinate combats all types of louse infestations when the manufacturer's directions are followed carefully. Because A-200 Pyrinate is accessible without prescription and highly effective, it accounts for 70 percent of all antilouse medication sales.

If a physician is consulted concerning lice, he will probably prescribe gamma benzene hexachloride as Kwell Cream, Lotion, or Shampoo. A single application of Kwell is usually effective, but may be repeated in one to four days if prescribed by the physician.

Other measures to help eliminate lice: boil and/or iron contaminated clothing, bedclothes, towels, and any other washables that are contaminated. Toilet seats, combs and brushes, and objects that can't be boiled can be cleansed with A-200 Pyrinate or Kwell Shampoo. Nits (eggs) attached to body hair should be picked off using a fine-tooth comb.

Scrupulous attention to personal hygiene is the best prophylaxis against pediculosis.

MARIJUANA

Synonyms: cannabis, grass, pot, and many more

Up to 20 million Americans have used marijuana at least once, and the drug is an integral part of the lives of many young individuals, the seemingly "square" as well as those on the fringes of society.

Marijuana is not a new drug, having been used as early as 2737 B.C. when Chinese Emperor Shen Nung recommended cannabis (the scientific name for marijuana) to treat "female weakness, gout, rheumatism, malaria, beriberi, and absent-mindedness." Through the centuries marijuana came to have fewer medicinal uses and found increasing favor as a social drug. Yet, as recently as 1950, a military study extolled the virtues of marijuana in the treatment of epilepsy, and a 1975 report tells how cannabis can relieve anxiety and reduce nausea in young cancer victims receiving chemotherapy.

Marijuana alters the mood, reportedly causing relaxation, a feeling of peacefulness, and a heightened sensitivity to surroundings. The pupils of the eye are contracted, and the eyelids may droop.

The chief problem that the reader of this book is likely to encounter is not in treating the victim of marijuana for overdosage, but in persuading youngsters that the use of marijuana is ill-advised.

The Case against Marijuana

The facts about marijuana should be carefully considered by all who contemplate its use:

- Marijuana is an illegal drug and its use not only

places the user outside the law but poses the danger of experimentation with this and possibly more potent drugs. A drug arrest can go "on the record," causing embarrassment or loss of a coveted opportunity in later life.

- Marijuana alters judgment and may lead to acts that would be avoided in a clearer frame of mind. Auto accidents, unwanted pregnancies, and many an ill-fated adventure have been linked to marijuana use.
- While marijuana is not defined as an addictive drug, the "pot" habit is hard to break. Habituation to marijuana can be as compelling as the alcohol or cigarette habits—which are perhaps more socially acceptable, but nevertheless difficult habit patterns to eliminate.
- The long-term safety of marijuana is in doubt. Current studies suggest that regular marijuana use may result in chromosome breakage, defective immunity against disease, chronic bronchitis, an increased risk of cancer, reduced sex drive, and a chronic lack of motivation.

All in all, there is little good to be said about marijuana and compelling reasons to avoid its use. Youngsters often say, "Your generation uses alcohol, and we prefer pot. What's the difference?"

Probably that's a good analogy, since alcoholism is a leading form of drug abuse that afflicts nine million Americans, and each year is implicated in 7,000 suicides; 25,000 traffic fatalities; up to three million arrests; and $15 billion in health care, time lost from work, and property damage. If marijuana is "no more harmful than alcohol," then heaven help us!

For more information about drug abuse, write to:

National Association for the Prevention of Narcotics Abuse
305 East 79th Street
New York, New York 10021

Narcotics Education
6830 Laurel Avenue
Washington, D.C. 20012

MASTITIS

Synonyms: inflammation of the breast, breast infection

Mastitis means inflammation of the breast and is a general term describing several ailments with different causes and cures: acute mastitis is a bacterial infection of the breast, while chronic mastitis describes painful, tender, but not infected lumps.

Acute Mastitis

Acute mastitis is a breast infection, usually caused by staphylococcus bacteria—the pus-forming germs responsible for so many infections, both superficial and deep. Although mastitis may strike the nonlactating breast, the most virulent infection occurs in the nursing mother, whose breast milk makes first-rate fodder for the infectious bacteria. The involved breast is hot, red, and swollen; fever is usually present and pain is severe.

The treatment of acute mastitis is similar to the therapy of bacterial infections elsewhere in the body. Antibiotics such as penicillin are prescribed, and the involved area is treated with hot packs applied for at least one hour four times daily. Nursing on the involved side is suspended until the infection clears.

Chronic Mastitis

Multiple breast lumps characterize chronic mastitis. The lumps form in response to the monthly rise and fall of female hormones as estrogens stimulate breast gland activity. The examining fingertip detects many small areas of fullness, with a scattered lump here and there; in advanced cases, the breast may feel like "a bag of marbles." The lumps of chronic mastitis are usually tender, in contrast to the malignant tumor that is most often pain-free in the early stages.

Chronic cystic mastitis is more worrisome than serious. Frequent checkups are necessary to detect the possible growth of any single lump, which would signal the need for removal.

The therapy of chronic mastitis may offer some relief, but is rarely curative. Warm compresses are helpful, particularly when pain occurs (most prominent in the week before the menstrual period). Oral contraceptives may alter the course of chronic cystic mastitis, by modifying the body's hormone balance. Ask your doctor for his recommendations.

It's possible that breast inflammation may be related to diethylstilbesterol (DES) fed to beef cattle, and a three-month trial of a beef-free diet may be warranted.

MEASLES

Synonyms: rubeola, red measles

Half a century ago Jerome K. Jerome penned the truism: "Love is like the measles; we all have to go through it."

Times have changed, and while most of us still "go through" love eventually, measles is no longer an inevitable event of childhood. The measles vaccine now enjoying widespread use has made the disease much less common than it was a generation ago, but the vaccine has rendered the detection of the sporadic case more difficult.

Measles is caused by a virus and is spread by "droplet infection," meaning that it is passed from person to person by coughing, sneezing, or personal contact. Following an incubation period of 10 to 14 days, measles first makes it presence known with fever, cough, and runny nose. The illness seems to be a common cold, but the wise parent examines the inside of the cheek for Koplik's spots—pinhead-size white spots surrounded by a pink-red halo. Next comes the typical rash of measles, beginning behind the ears or on the neck and spreading to involve the entire body. Fever above 102°F is the rule, and the eyes are a telltale bright red.

The acute disease lasts about a week, with the fever subsiding and the rash fading gradually. It's time to return to school when the skin and eyes are clear, the cough is gone, the appetite has returned to normal, and the child seems fit in all ways.

Treating and Preventing Measles

Aspirin, bed rest, and fluids are the backbone of measles treatment. Aspirin in given for fever, in a dose of one grain per year of age (up to a maximum of 10 grains) every six to eight hours if fever is present. Bed rest allows the body to marshal its full resources to fight the infection, and extra fluids are taken to prevent dehydration.

Mothers often wonder if the room should be kept dark to protect the eyes. Although the youngster may complain that bright lights are annoying, light in the room, or even reading, will cause no ocular damage.

Measles should be prevented rather than treated, and the measles vaccination campaign aims to confer "herd immunity," meaning that so many individuals would have natural or acquired immunity that an epidemic couldn't get started, and the few susceptible children escape exposure to the disease. Measles virus vaccine, live (Attenuvax), should be given to all children one year of age or older if they have not already had measles and if there is no contraindication to measles vaccination such as leukemia or lymphoma, active tuberculosis, allergy to eggs, an acute infection, or current treatment with cortisone, anticancer drugs, or x-ray therapy.

Some children receiving live measles vaccine will suffer a fever and/or rash 5 to 12 days after the injection, but severe reactions are uncommon. Live measles vaccination confers long-lasting immunity to 97 percent of those inoculated, with the remaining 3 percent still at risk, but hopefully protected by herd immunity.

The live measles vaccine offers no protection if given after exposure to the disease, and in this instance the doctor may advise measles-immune human globulin for short-term protection. A large dose may prevent the manifestations of measles, while a smaller injection modifies the course of the illness. The use of measles-immune human globulin is particularly indicated when the disease threatens nonimmune infants or unprotected individuals sick with other illnesses. Two or more months after receiving temporary protection with measles-immune human globulin, the live measues vaccine should be given.

MENIERE'S DISEASE

A whirling dizziness called vertigo, a ringing in the ears called tinnitus, and impaired hearing characterize Meniere's disease—an uncommon chronic disorder of the inner ear. Symptoms may wax and wane, perhaps becoming worse during times of colds and flu or when anxious, only to diminish during periods of mental and physical well-being.

Managing Meniere's Disease

The elimination of caffeine-containing beverages and tobacco is a first in therapy. A low-fluid diet may help, since Meniere's disease is often related to excessive fluid in the balance canals of the inner ear, and dietary salt restriction helps achieve a lower inner ear fluid pressure.

More aggressive therapy requires a prescription, and the doctor may recommend an antihistamine such as meclizine (Bonine) or dimenhydrinate (Dramamine) to control vertigo. Sometimes a diuretic such as hydrochlorothiazide (Esidrex) is prescribed, usually taken with orange juice to prevent potassium depletion. In addition, Meniere's disease sufferers should follow the hints to help avoid vertigo described under Labyrinthitis (page 192).

MENINGITIS

Synonyms: cerebrospinal meningitis, spinal meningitis

Meningitis poses a danger to life and threatens brain function in those who survive. Several different bacteria can cause meningitis including the meningococcus, Hemophilus influenza bacilli, and others. The H. influenza meningitis usually strikes young children, while meningococcal meningitis may occur at any age. A hemorrhagic rash (bleeding spots under the skin) may occur with meningococcal meningitis, while H. influenza meningitis often follows a common cold or ear infection.

By far, the most important aspect of self-help care is recognition of possible meningitis, followed by an immediate call to the physician. Prompt therapy with high doses of antibiotics can be lifesaving, and unnecessary delay can result in needless complications.

Five cardinal symptoms characterize meningitis:

- Stiffness of the neck is a hallmark. We're not discussing the mild neck discomfort and general achiness of a viral flu, but rather a true neck rigidity that makes it impossible for the patient to touch his chin to his chest.
- High fever accompanies meningitis, but don't be lulled into complacency by a temporary temperature drop. If linked with the other symptoms noted here, high fever should suggest possible meningitis.
- Agonizing headache characterizes infection of the meningeal lining of the brain. The headache may be in the forehead, the back of the head, or involve the whole head. No matter; whatever its location, an exceptionally severe headache accompanied by fever and other signs of acute illness can be the tip-off to an early meningitis.
- Impaired consciousness is a danger signal, and the youngster or adult who becomes poorly responsive, who fails to respond to speech or even to pain, should be examined by the doctor immediately.
- Weakness of muscles, such as poor convergence of the eyes, impaired walking, or other evidence of poor muscle function, might be caused by meningitis, if associated with fever or other symptoms of infection.

Meningitis-causing bacteria multiply rapidly. Minutes and hours count! If confronted with one or more of the five meningitis symptoms listed above, call the physician or go to the hospital without delay.

MENOPAUSE

Synonyms: climacteric, change of life

At some time between ages 40 and 55 the average woman sees menstrual flow cease, perhaps followed a few months later by periodic hot flushes. During these same years, most women undergo an upheaval in their lives: children depart for school, jobs, or marriage; her husband may communicate dissatisfaction with work or even with their marriage; and the woman herself may undertake an agonizing reappraisal of her life's goals and accomplishments. Altogether, these phenomena are called the menopause—the change of life.

Irritability, apathy, depression—they're all symptoms attributed to the menopause, and during the fifth decade of life most mood changes and physical symptoms are attributed to the change of life.

In point of fact, the absence of menstrual flow and the onset of hot flashes are the only physical manifestations unique to the climacteric. Fatigue, apathy, joint pains, headaches, and all the rest may be linked to emotional tension, aging, or some specific illness, but should not necessarily be blamed upon the lower levels of ovarian hormones that characterize the menopause.

What to Do about Menopause

Positive thinking can banish many supposed menopausal woes, while other physical complaints may respond to prescribed medication. Here are the facts:

- Realize that anxiety or depression occurring during this time often has emotional origins, and is not always attributable to a hormone deficiency. Seek psychological causes for mood changes and attack problems squarely. If necessary, make an appointment for professional counseling, perhaps supplemented by a mild tranquilizer.
- Hot flushes are caused by low ovarian hormone levels. Female hormones are controlled by blood substances called chorionic gonadotropins manufactured in the pituitary. Chorionic gonadotropins have two properties: they increase the production of ovarian hormones and they cause circulatory instability seen as hot flushes. During the reproductive years, gonadotropins had the job of maintaining adequate hormone levels in the blood. When hormone levels fall during the menopause, the pituitary produces large quantities of chorionic gonadotropins for the following few years in a vain effort to coax more hormones from the

failing ovaries. But all that is achieved is the production of hot flushes, occurring at unpredictable times. Fortunately, hot flushes respond to hormone therapy, and the doctor often prescribes conjugated equine estrogens as Premarin Tablets taken 21 or perhaps 25 days each month.

- Supplementary hormone tablets can also help hold back the hands of time, slowing many of the changes of aging that are accelerated after the menopause, including wrinkling of the skin and softening of the bones. But a word of caution: recently released studies indicate that estrogen tablets may increase the risk of uterine endometrial cancer and and can raise the risk of heart attack—in turn related to higher triglyceride and blood pressure levels.

- Yes, you can get pregnant during the menopause. Here and there, ovulation occurs and if the released egg has the good (or bad, depending on your outlook) fortune to meet a wayward sperm, fertilization can occur. When are you really safe? My advice is this: The woman who has gone two years without a menstrual period is 99.99 percent safe. If in doubt, see Contraception on page 82.

One by one, the traditional menopausal myths are being exploded. For every woman whose change-of-life years brings apathy and depression, there are three who discover that the middle years—with lessened parental responsibilities, diminished household duties, increasing opportunities in all phases of business and society, and the possibility of sex without worries about contraception—can be her best ever.

The Male Menopause

Of course it's a misnomer, since menopause means cessation of the menses, yet men sometimes suffer change-of-life symptoms. Most notable are lassitude, despondency, and a waning sexual interest and performance.

Here and there you find an individual with physical disease to explain the symptoms—perhaps diabetes, alcoholism, pernicious anemia, premature arteriosclerosis, or even possibly multiple sclerosis. But the vast majority of men suffering change-of-life symptoms can attribute their complaints to psychological causes. One common source is the discontent of middle age: the victim is unhappy with his job, his family, and himself. Often he seeks to solve his problem by impulsive action, seeking a job change, divorce, or a "new personality." Early symptoms may be growing a mustache or beard, trading the family station wagon for a sports car, or making passes at girls half his age. In the end, efforts to effect sweeping changes almost always fail, as divorce is followed by remarriage to a wife who's the carbon copy of the first (yet now the husband must support two households) or he quits one job to take another only to find the same tedium he had hoped to escape.

A special problem of Mr. Middle Age is the failure fantasy. For decades, he's promised himself that by age 50 he would be a success—perhaps vice president, a published writer, plant foreman, or chief of staff. Then the fortieth or even fiftieth birthday comes and goes, and suddenly there is the realization that he'll never make it. His lifelong goals are beyond his grasp, and probably despite succeeding at his job, not to mention providing for his family, he sees himself a failure during middle age.

There's no medicine to help this man. Hormones, vitamins, tonics, and all the rest cannot splint his fractured ego or bolster his lagging vitality. What's needed is a realistic self-appraisal, reevaluating goals, and placing a true value on accomplishments. When the man in his change-of-life apathy makes an objective evaluation of his life, he almost always finds that assets exceed liabilities by a wide margin. And the male menopause becomes more fantasy than fact.

MENSTRUAL DISORDERS

Between the onset of menstrual flow (menarche) and its cessation (menopause), most women have a menstrual period each lunar month. The monthly menstrual flow is regulated by the female hormones—estrogen and progesterone—as they rise, causing growth of the cells lining the uterus, then fall when fertilization fails to occur. Next comes the loss of the uterine lining cells in the form of the menses, once described as the uterus "weeping for the pregnancy that might have been."

The cyclic rise and fall of hormones is usually orderly, yet is influenced by so many factors that it's a wonder that menstrual flow occurs as regularly as it does. The following is a list of the disorders of menstruation and what you should know about them:

- Amenorrhea means an absent or "skipped" period. During the child-bearing years, pregnancy must always be considered, and a pregnancy test may provide the answer
- Cryptomenorrhea means hidden menstrual flow. It is a problem found in young girls as the flow of her first menstrual periods becomes trapped behind an intact hymen. The rising pressure of menstrual blood causes an intense discomfort, immediately relieved when the physician perforates the hymenal membrane.
- Delayed menarche refers to a late onset of menstrual periods. There will probably also be slow development of breast tissue and adult hair distribution. A family tendency toward late development is often common, and little concern is warranted until the mid-teens.
- Dysmenorrhea is the medical term for menstrual cramps, caused by swelling in the pelvic tissues, contraction of uterine muscle, and perhaps an unhealthy attitude toward menstruation. Sometimes it helps to take a diuretic beginning the week before the menstrual period is due. Hot baths or a heating pad applied to the abdomen may bring temporary relief. Green leafy vegetables are time-honored folk remedies for menstrual cramps, and naturalists recommend eating increased amounts of cabbage, lettuce, and parsley before and during the menstrual period. The sporadic use of aspirin is permitted, but menstrual cramps demanding stronger analgesics suggest the need for a medical examination. Sometimes the doctor will prescribe oral contraceptives—menstrual cramps are related to ovulation, and often fade when oral contraceptives suspend the monthly release of an egg from the ovary.
- Menorrhagia is flooding, the monthly loss of excessive blood with the menstrual period. Anemia may result, and examination is needed to rule out the possibility of cancer or a uterine fibroid tumor.

- Metrorrhagia is bleeding between periods, with day-by-day spotting, perhaps worse following sexual intercourse. A common cause is a low-dose oral contraceptive, and a stronger pill usually solves the problem. If metrorrhagia is persistent, examination is mandatory since possible causes include a cervical polyp, uterine fibroids, or malignancy.
- Mittelschmerz comes from the German word meaning pain in the middle of the cycle. The discomfort is related to release of the egg (ovulation) and is usually described as sharp and brief. It's important that mittelschmerz be recognized for what it is, since right-sided pain may be confused with acute appendicitis.
- Oligomenorrhea means reduced menstrual flow, common with oral contraceptives, normal at the time of the menopause, but sometimes associated with infertility.
- Premenstrual tension is a "bitchy" feeling during the week before the menstrual period. Fluid retention is a major factor, and women often complain of swelling of the feet and fingers. The emotional irritability is related to fluid pressure on the brain, and relief often follows a morning diuretic tablet such as hydrochlorothiazide (Esidrex) plus restriction of dietary salt.

Menstrual disorders are magnified, and sometimes caused, by improper attitudes toward the monthly menstrual cycle. Menstruation is a normal female function and should not be described by disease-related terms such as "unwell" or "curse" or "sickness." When the young girl shows early breast budding and the emergence of an adult hair distribution, the menstrual flow can't be far behind, and she should be psychologically prepared. Discuss menstruation with her, explaining how the cycle prepares her body to have a baby, and that the menstrual flow discharges this preparation—to be followed by another cycle next month. Encourage her to be proud of her femininity and her monthly evidence of fertility.

Since the monthly menstrual flow is a normal function, a small amount of discomfort should be tolerable without undue apprehension, and with a minimal use of analgesics. Girls should not stay home from school or significantly change their routine during the menstrual period. A daily bath or shower is encouraged, but the use of feminine hygiene sprays is unnecessary.

I'm often asked about the use of vaginal tampons. Certainly they are an accepted institution, and there is no reason why the mature teen-age girl cannot use an intravaginal tampon. My only reservation is this: when any object is left inside a body cavity, a "foreign body" reaction begins, and infection often follows. In office practice, young women with recurrent vaginal infections may attain long-lasting relief only when they cease the use of intravaginal tampons.

MOLES

Synonyms: nevus, nevi

We all have moles, some a few, others more. The usual nevus is a harmless "beauty mark" or blemish—depending upon your frame of mind—and moles are removed for two reasons: to improve the patient's cosmetic appearance or because there is a worry about malignant change.

Not all moles can be removed, or America's physicians would be employed full-time removing harmless skin lesions. Judgement is needed, and there are guidelines to help decide if a mole should be surgically excised:

- Remove any mole that is repeatedly inflamed, particularly if scabbing or bleeding occur.
- Remove moles subject to repeated chafing, such as those in the belt, bra, or collar lines. Also removed should be any mole repeatedly nicked while shaving.
- Moles on the palms of the hand and soles of the feet have an increased malignant potential and are usually removed.
- Any mole that enlarges or shows a spread in pigmentation should be excised.
- Remove any nevus that you and your doctor decide is questionable for any reason.
- Elective removal may be recommended for facial moles that constitute major cosmetic defects.

Most moles are removed surgically, taking an ellipse of skin, after which the edges are stitched together (see Figure

21). The excised mole is examined in the laboratory for suspected malignant change. A scar will result following removal of any mole, and appearance will depend upon the skill of the surgeon, the size of the mole, and the site on the body; the removal of facial moles results in more cosmetically acceptable scarring than excision of moles from thick-skinned areas such as the shoulders and back.

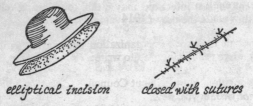

elliptical incision   closed with sutures

FIGURE 21. *Surgical removal of a mole.*

MONGOLISM

Synonym: Down's syndrome

Mongolism is caused by an abnormality of chromosomes in the body cells. The incidence is about one in every 600 births but rises with maternal age, so that for the 40-year-old expectant mother the risk is about one in 100 births.

This birth defect can be detected at 14 to 16 weeks of pregnancy by a procedure called amniocentesis: a needle is inserted in the womb and fetal cells are withdrawn and microscopically examined. At this point the affected pregnancy can legally be terminated by abortion.

The Mongoloid individual is trainable and pleasant, but often has a heart defect and is prone to infection. Most don't survive past the teen-age years.

A book for professionals and parents published in 1975 discusses the cause, course, and treatment of Down's syndrome, the use of 5-hydroxytryptophane, employment training, and sexuality of the mentally retarded. Ask your bookseller to order *Down's Syndrome (Mongolism): Research, Prevention, and Management,* edited by Richard Koch, M.D., and Felix F. de la Cruz, M.D. (Brunner/Mazel, New York). Information on Mongolism can be obtained from:

The National Foundation-March of Dimes
P. O. Box 2000
White Plains, New York 10602

National Institute for Mental Health
Information Office
Bethesda, Maryland 20014

Atlhough no national organization deals solely with Mongolism, there is a local group to write:

Mongoloid Development Council
307 Bender Avenue
Roselle Park, New Jersey 07204
Telephone: (201) 241-6137

MOTION SICKNESS

Synonym: carsickness

Motion sickness may occur when riding in any vehicle—automobile, boat, or airplane. Nausea, often accompanied by vomiting, is the chief symptom, although patients may also describe lightheadedness and a cold clammy sensation of the skin. The greater the undulating motion of the vehicle, the more likely the onset of motion sickness.

What to Do about Motion Sickness

Susceptible individuals should anticipate problems and plan ahead. Nothing should be taken by mouth within one hour of beginning a trip. If riding in an airplane, say "No, thanks" to the stewardess' offer of alcoholic beverages, and, when traveling by car, try to avoid snacks until you have reached your destination.

Medication can help, and the faithful standby of motion sickness sufferers has been the antihistamine. Nonprescription dimenhydrinate (Dramamine) and meclizine (Bonine) are most often used, helping prevent the nausea and vomiting of motion sickness. The major side effect is drowsiness, which can sometimes be avoided by careful dose adjustment.

Time heals many things, including motion sickness. Some individuals have overcome their problem by taking repeated automobile trips or ocean voyages, squarely facing their affliction and overcoming it.

MOUTH BREATHING

The mouth breather lives with slack jaw, lower lip hanging open, and respiratory passages irritated by tiny particles that should be filtered by nasal hair. The penalty for chronic mouth breathing is often gum disease, dental caries, bad breath, morning cough, and an increased incidence of respiratory infections.

Overcoming Mouth Breathing

The habitual mouth breather needs no more therapy than constant awareness that the lips should be kept closed and that breathing should be through the nose. It may take months to break old habits, and nocturnal mouth breathing during sleep is especially hard to overcome.

Nasal obstruction and/or enlarged adenoids may cause obligatory mouth breathing, as narrow nasopharyngeal passages prohibit normal breathing. Surgical correction of a deviated septum, excision of a nasal polyp, or removal of massive adenoids may restore normal breathing.

Allergy is a common offender, and alleviation of allergic symptoms—whether through avoidance, antihistamines, or injections—may overcome mouth breathing and restore normal respiration (see Hay Fever).

MULTIPLE MYELOMA

Synonym: plasma cell myeloma

Multiple myeloma is a neoplastic disease characterized by large numbers of plasma cells—one of the several types of cells found in normal blood. When the number of plasma cells reaches huge levels, symptoms begin. Islands of plasma cells in the bone marrow may weaken the supporting structure and cause fractures, and plasma cells in kidney tissues cause urinary abnormalities. Anemia is common as neoplastic cells crowd out normal red and white blood cells, and the disease progresses to renal failure, increased susceptibility to infection, and fatal termination.

Detecting multiple myeloma can be a challenge. It is not a common disorder, but should be kept in mind whenever there is recurrent and persistent bone pain, particularly severe backache for which no cause is evident.

Once his suspicions have been aroused, the doctor will make the diagnosis on the basis of blood tests, bone biopsy, or bone marrow examination.

Treatment may involve melphalan (Alkeran) or cyclophosphamide (Cytoxan).

MULTIPLE SCLEROSIS

Synonyms: MS, disseminated sclerosis

An estimated half million Americans suffer multiple sclerosis, a disorder of the nervous system most common in young adults. The disease is more common in temperate than in subtropical climates, strikes women more often than men, and may show a family pattern.

The symptoms of multiple sclerosis are kaleidoscopic. Generations of medical students have memorized Charcot's triad of symptoms found in many cases: nystagmus (a rapid motion of the eye when looking to the side), an intention tremor (shaking of the hand when initiating a motion), and scanning speech (hesitant speech lacking accents and rhythm). Early symptoms are usually elusive, and may include brief episodes of double vision, impaired memory, spells of dizziness, and momentary weakness of one or more extremities.

The disease progresses in an episodic fashion, with flare-ups punctuating relatively symptom-free intervals during the early years. In time, perhaps over a 10 to 15-year span, symptom-free intervals disappear and chronic disability is the rule, with occasional flare-ups requiring intensive therapy.

Treatment

There is no cure for MS. Still, much can be done. Physical therapy is important, and affected extremities should receive active and passive exercises two or three times daily, building strength and retaining full range of motion. A limb weakened by MS can be strengthened by braces, and walking may be aided by Canadian crutches, a cane, or walker.

Muscle spasm is often a problem, and the doctor may prescribe diazepam (Valium) or the newer dantrolene (Dantrium). Acute flare-ups often respond to cortisone therapy.

Mercifully, the multiple sclerosis victim usually has a mild euphoria that is characteristic of the disease and helps prevent depression.

If you or someone in your family has MS, contact the National Multiple Sclerosis Society, 257 Park Avenue South, New York, New York 10010, and learn the address of the local MS chapter near you. Here you may find available aids for daily living such as walkers, wheelchairs, and special beds, as well as counseling and guidance in obtaining physical therapy, occupational therapy, social services, and visiting nurses.

MUMPS

Synonym: epidemic parotitis

Mumps is another of the childhood diseases that, like measles, need never occur. Boys, particularly, should receive protection against mumps, since mumps occurring in the postpubertal male can cause severe inflammation of the testes and may result in sterility.

Although the most striking manifestation of mumps is the enlargement of the salivary glands overlying the mandible (lower jaw), mumps is a general infection that also causes fever, loss of appetite, headache, lassitude, and often abdominal pain. The diagnosis of mumps can be elusive, with many mothers insisting that their youngsters had mumps when, in fact, the child has suffered only an episode of swollen glands in the neck that mimicked mumps.

There is no cure for mumps, and therapy is directed toward relief of symptoms. Aspirin is given for fever and pain, and a soft, bland diet is provided, avoiding citrus juices that may provoke discomfort in the salivary gland. Bed rest is advised during the acute stage of the disease, with return to school allowed only after all symptoms have subsided.

Mumps therapy includes keeping an eye out for complications: mumps orchitis (inflammation of the testicle) causes swelling and pain of the scrotum in up to 25 percent of postpubertal males. Females may suffer oophoritis—an inflammation of the ovaries, signaled by pain in the left or right quadrant of the abdomen. A more ominous complication is mumps encephalitis, which causes headache, restlessness, drowsiness, and perhaps a stiff neck, with mental confusion. If any of these complications are suspected, call the doctor immediately.

Mumps can be prevented by administration of the live mumps virus vaccine (Mumpsvax). A single dose of the vaccine provides long-term protection for approximately 97 percent of children and 93 percent of adults. Although an occasional individual suffers fever and/or parotid gland discomfort following the vaccine, the incidence of side effects is very low and live mumps virus vaccine should be given to all adults and children over one year of age who have not had mumps, and who do not have a contraindication to vaccination such as pregnancy; allergy to eggs or to neomycin; blood disorders including leukemia, a deficiency of gamma globulin, or an active infection; or are undergoing treatment with cortisone, anticancer drugs, or x-ray therapy. Live mumps virus vaccine must be given prior to exposure to the disease, and once a susceptible postpubertal adult male has come in contact with the disease, he can receive short-term protection by an injection of mumps-hyperimmune gamma globulin.

MUSCULAR DYSTROPHY

Muscular dystrophy is an uncommon genetic disorder chiefly striking children and characterized by progressive muscle weakness. The leg muscles are usually involved, causing a waddling gait and a curious manner of arising by "climbing up one's legs."

The medical treatment of muscular dystrophy is disappointing and progressive paralysis is the common outcome. Many medications have been prescribed including vitamin E, inositol, amino acid and protein substances, but none has proved to be beneficial. If muscle tightness is a problem, the physician may prescribe quinine tablets and muscle wasting may be countered with body-building androgenic hormones.

Self-help therapy of muscular dystrophy is as follows: Obesity must be avoided since each extra pound places a burden on already weakened muscle. Activity is encouraged and excessive bedrest avoided. In all spheres, the muscular dystrophy patient should strive to maintain the most normal life possible within the limitations imposed by his disease.

Self-help information plus facts concerning special hospitals (and possible funds available) may be obtained by writing to:

Muscular Dystrophy Association of America
1790 Broadway
New York, New York 10019

MUSHROOM POISONING

Most mushroom poisoning in America is caused by Amanita mushrooms that cause vomiting, diarrhea, nausea, and abdominal pain, perhaps associated with salivation, perspiration, shortness of breath, excitability, and confusion. Symptoms begin about six hours after eating the poisonous mushrooms.

It's easy to avoid mushroom poisonings; eat only commercially prepared mushrooms. It's not safe for amateurs to attempt identification of the poisonous and nonpoisonous varieties.

If the vomiting, diarrhea, and cramps characteristic of food poisoning begin, consider the possibility of mushroom poisoning. If the ingestion of toxic mushrooms is suspected, see the doctor. He may prescribe sedatives to calm anxiety, and perhaps atropine to combat the muscarine poison present in some mushrooms.

MYASTHENIA GRAVIS

An uncommon disorder, myasthenia gravis is a pathological weakness of muscles, first noted as drooping eyelids when fatigued. Later symptoms may be double vision due to weak eye muscles, with impaired speech and swallowing.

The disease may occur at any age, but usually involves young individuals, whose symptoms become worse as a result of fatigue, excitement, infection, and the use of alcohol.

When faced with an individual whose eyelids droop, and whose voice may "run out of steam" at the end of a sentence or two, the doctor thinks: "Could this patient have myasthenia gravis?"

Confirmatory tests use drugs such as neostigmine (Prostigmin) or edrophonium chloride (Tensilon).

The individual with myasthenia gravis must avoid such precipitating factors as strong laxatives, high enemas, alcohol use, and certain drugs including quinine, quinidine, curare, morphine, ether, and chloroform.

For further information write:

The Myasthenia Gravis Foundation
2 East 103rd Street
New York, New York 10029

NARCOTIC ABUSE

Synonyms: drug abuse, drug addiction

From the Greek *narkos*, meaning sleep, comes the name of the broad class of drugs causing altered consciousness and sharing a pernicious propensity for addiction. Commonly abused narcotics include heroin, morphine, meperidine (Demerol), codeine, paregoric, and methadone—all derived from or sharing properties with the opium poppy.

Most commonly abused is heroin—admittedly a first-rate analgesic whose use is no longer permitted in America because of the dangers of addiction. Less potent morphine and meperidine have a considerable addiction potential, and are often prescribed for the relief of severe pain. Methadone is a favorite drug to "treat" narcotics addiction, although oral administration of it has led some to discount its potential for addiction, and the distribution of methadone in fruit juice has led to unwitting ingestion by innocent household members. Codeine is a commonly prescribed analgesic and a component of many cough preparations, while paregoric is a time-honored remedy for diarrhea.

Certain signs and symptoms characterize the narcotics user. When under the influence of a narcotic drug, the individual may exhibit poor attentiveness and have small, constricted pupils. Needle marks may be seen on the arms. With overdosage comes impaired consciousness that may lead to coma, slow breathing, and a falling blood pressure. Death due to narcotic abuse may follow blood poisoning, pneumonia occurring during coma, or the overdose ("OD") following the injection of an uncut dose of drugs.

Dealing with Narcotic Abuse

Narcotics experts view drug use as a symptom—not a disease. The individual turns to drugs due to anxiety, frustration, depression, isolation, and/or other causes of emotional upheaval. A broken home, peer pressure, and a lack of opportunity for achievement are common factors. Attempts to deal with drug use as an isolated problem are futile (as witnessed by the distressing failure rate following forced withdrawal in the institutions of the past generation) and therapy must include psychological counseling, social readjustment, and vocational rehabilitation.

The first step in dealing with drug abuse is to recognize its presence. Parents should tune in to symptoms of poor school work, a sudden disinterest in after-school activities, and a withdrawal from friends and family. And young people must be cognizant of the dangers of experimentation with hardcore drugs whose "occasional" use can expand into an all-consuming addiction.

When drugs present a problem, seek help. Most communities now have drug-control programs, led by counselors with up-to-date training. In fact, many community drug counselors are ex-addicts tuned in to the problem of narcotic abuse, and these individuals can guide the youngster into programs that encourage drug abstinence while supporting his ego and filling psychological needs with creative outlets. Methadone therapy has been the subject of controversy, but remains a useful tool when administered by skilled therapists and when coupled with intensive counseling and rehabilitation.

Only when the individual's psychological needs are met by socially acceptable alternatives, such as a job and family, can the drug problem be pronounced cured.

For further information write to:

Addicts Anonymous
Box 2000
Lexington, Kentucky 40507

International Federation for Narcotic Education
918 F Street, N. W.
Washington, D.C. 20004

Narcotics Education
6830 Laurel Avenue
Washington, D.C. 20012

National Association for the Prevention of Addiction to Narcotics (NAPAN)
250 West 57th Street
New York, New York 10019

NEUROPATHY

Synonyms: nerve degeneration, neuralgia, neuritis

A disorder of one or more of the nerves of the body is called a neuropathy, which may be described as an inflammation (neuritis) that may or may not cause pain (neuralgia). Many types of neuropathy occur, and the cure is related to the cause:

- Trigeminal neuralgia, also called tic douloureux, is an inflammation of the fifth cranial nerve that causes severe pain of one side of the face. The cause is occasionally a dental problem, and a consultation with the dentist is worthwhile. But usually the cause is elusive, and treatment may include analgesics such as propoxyphene (Darvon), specific medication such as carbamazepine (Tegretol), or perhaps surgical destruction of a portion of the nerve.

- Facial paralysis, known as Bell's palsy (*q.v.*), follows damage to the seventh cranial nerve that controls the muscles of the face. The mouth is pulled to the unaffected side, there is difficulty in closing the eye, and a weakness of the muscle prevents wrinkling of the forehead. Sometimes the cause is an ear infection injuring the seventh nerve as it passes adjacent to the ear structures. The doctor may prescribe cortisone compounds, along with physical therapy for the muscles and nerves. Most, but not all, victims recover spontaneously after a few months.
- Erb's paralysis is a withered arm caused by damage to the brachial nerve plexus above the collarbone. Birth injury is the usual cause and exercise to strengthen the remaining muscle is the only therapy.
- Wrist-drop occurs when there is damage to the nerve supplying the forearm muscles. Sometimes the cause is lead poisoning, and a blood test should be done.
- Sciatica is an inflammation of the sciatic nerve, often beginning as a slipped lower spinal disc presses upon nerve fibers leaving the spinal column. Rest, local applications of heat, and time bring relief in many patients, although surgery to remove the protruding disc is often necessary.
- Meralgia paresthetica causes a tingling discomfort along the outer thigh. A common cause is a tight girdle or a low-slung belt (such as a policeman's gunbelt), causing pressure on a sensory nerve. Release the pressure and the symptoms disappear.
- Ulnar nerve palsy causes numbness and weakness of the fourth and fifth fingers, and usually follows damage to the ulnar nerve in the elbow. An injured or even fractured elbow is a common cause, although even a few hours of sustained pressure on the elbow can cause symptoms that will last for weeks or months.
- Foot-drop follows injury to the peroneal nerve that curves around the upper end of the fibula near the knee. The thin individual who sits for long hours with

one leg crossed over the other (such as a tailor) may bruise the peroneal nerve and suffer a foot-drop, walking with a "steppage gait" as the foot-drop requires high-stepping to avoid dragging the foot.

Neuropathies can occur with many diseases, including diabetes, alcoholism, and pernicious anemia (all discussed elsewhere in this book). One or more extremities may be involved, and the patient often describes sensations of tingling, burning, and pain, sometimes relieved when the causative disease is discovered and controlled.

NEUROSIS

Synonym: psychoneurosis

The member of the neurotic population may console himself with the knowledge that his chronic disorder places him among the majority of the population; that his difficulties arise from a common wellspring of the human condition; and that the dynamism of the neurosis may contribute energy to his particular personality or genius.

David Seegal
Journal of the American Medical
Association 182: 1031 (1962)

Those who channel their neurotic energy into worthwhile channels are among our most productive citizens, while others are overwhelmed by neurotic symptoms and spend their days in doctors' offices.

The following are but some of the common neuroses:

- Anxiety neurosis is as common as ants at a picnic, afflicting millions of Americans who live their lives in constant, yet ill-defined dread. This ubiquitous disorder is discussed in detail on page 23.
- Compulsions and obsessions describe the overwhelming urge to perform senseless acts and pointless rituals. Harmless compulsions may be called habits—hanging the overcoat on the same hook each

evening, washing clothes on Monday instead of Tuesday, or reaching for a cigarette when the telephone rings. But other compulsions may interfere with the victim's daily activities and health—smoking two packs of cigarettes a day, washing the hands every few minutes, gambling away the paycheck each week, or overeating to obesity.

- Conversion hysteria occurs when neurotic anxiety is transferred to one area of the body. A prime example is stage fright, occurring as an anxious individual suffers difficulty breathing and inability to speak when faced with a microphone and audience. Other examples include muscle tics, hysterical paralysis of one or more extremities, or the inability to take a deep breath (hyperventilation).

- Neurasthenia means weakness of the nerves, and describes an all-consuming chronic fatigue. Exhaustive diagnostic studies reveal no physical abnormality, although the blood pressure may be slightly low, the reflexes a trifle sluggish, and appetite impaired, and the energy level almost zero.

- Depression, discussed in more detail on page 95, is a black mood of apathy and hopelessness often due to some type of loss—death of a loved one, divorce, business failure, or loss of a job. Sometimes, however, no cause is apparent. Depression is cyclic, and the outlook is best when a clear-cut cause is correctable.

- Phobias are unreasonable fears, perhaps linked to a traumatic incident in the past. Common are fears of closed places (claustophobia), high places (acrophobia), malignancy (cancerophobia), darkness (nyctophobia), and the sight of blood (hemophobia).

Most of us suffer one or more minor neurotic symptoms. We recognize our problems for what they are and cope with them. But when psychoneurotic complaints interfere with our jobs, families, and health, it's time for treatment.

Overcoming Psychoneurosis

Self-help treatment of psychoneurosis concerns gaining insight into the disorder, and learning to cope with neurotic tendencies by facing them head-on.

Choose a quiet afternoon to analyze your problem with pencil and paper. First list all symptoms that you think are caused by your neurosis. Perhaps your list will include sleeplessness, loss of appetite, dry cracked hands due to frequent hand-washing, palpitation when faced with responsibility or public speaking, an apparent addiction to chocolate cake, or the fear that you suffer brain cancer.

Next, write down how these symptoms interfere with your daily life. The salesman who fears meeting strangers may find his job in jeopardy. The smoking athlete won't be on the team for long. And the tired housewife never seems to get the housework done.

Step three is analysis. Write down what you think may be contributing to the neurosis. Compulsive overeaters may, as teenagers, have turned to the refrigerator when anxiety threatened. A fear of heights may be traced to a childhood mishap, or neurasthenia may be the only way the wife can gain her husband's attention and sympathy.

Discuss your list and analysis with the doctor, or perhaps with a psychotherapist or minister. The discussion may bring out points that you hadn't considered, and an objective third party can contribute helpful suggestions. Finally, plan a program for dealing with the neurosis. Stage fright may be overcome by joining a public-speaking class or club. A morbid fear of closed spaces may respond to a structured program of short periods of controlled confinement in tight quarters, eventually culminating in the much-feared elevator ride. Neurasthenia may vanish following a program of physical exercise. Confronting the cause of fear can have the same effect as taking allergy injections: bit by bit, the mind's response to the dreaded stimulus is desensitized.

There are pitfalls in coping with neurosis, and the individual must be wary of cure-all remedies, untrained counselors, and overenthusiastic attempts to exorcise the neurosis. Here's a list of DONT'S for the neurotic:

- Don't blame all symptoms on the neurosis. Even the neurotic can suffer physical illness.
- Don't hesitate to seek another opinion if you seem at odds with a doctor or psychotherapist. Even counselors have their hang-ups, and don't let Doc substitute his neuroses for yours.
- Don't allow yourself to act out your neurosis on the

job or at home, snapping at co-workers or magnifying domestic difficulties.

- Don't waste good money on tonics that are probably merely vitamins and minerals in an alcohol base. These usually have little more than placebo value.
- Don't take medicine unless it's prescribed by the physician, and then his directions should be followed to the letter.
- Read *I'm O.K.—You're O.K.* by Thomas A. Harris (Harper & Row, New York), telling how to give and get love and approval, rejection and disapproval.
- Call the doctor if neurotic symptoms blight your life despite self-analysis and an honest effort to lick your problems. Describe your urges and anxieties honestly.

NIGHT SWEATS

The victim of night sweats awakes from sleep with his bed-clothes drenched by perspiration. Beads of sweat break out on all areas of the body. Night sweats, uncommon in young persons, usually involve middle-aged or older individuals.

The cause of night sweats is often obscure. Sometimes the answer is as easy as an overheated bedroom or too many blankets; sometimes opening a window to improve ventilation allows restful slumber. But be wary: night sweats, like fever, can be a symptom of more serious disease. In days gone by, doctors often linked night sweats with tuberculosis. Today, tuberculosis is less common, but night sweats may be a symptom of chronic infection, undetected malignancy, or perhaps a disorder of metabolism.

If night sweats are a chronic problem, particularly if they have begun in recent weeks or months, see the doctor for a thorough diagnostic examination.

NOSEBLEED

Synonyms: epistaxis, bloody nose
Nosebleeds occur for many reasons, including nasal congestion of a head cold, high blood pressure, impaired blood

clotting, and nocturnal nose-picking by restless youngsters. Most nosebleeds originate on the middle wall of the nose near the opening of the nostrils (see Figure 22), and bleeding originating in this area is predominantly one-sided. Firm pressure of the thumb against the bleeding should arrest the nosebleed if pressure is held long enough. Squeeze firmly for 15 minutes; don't let up every few seconds to see if bleeding has ceased. Remain sitting rather than lying down, thus lowering the blood pressure slightly. Most nosebleeds stop with simple pressure. However, recurrent bleeding may require packing or cautery by the doctor.

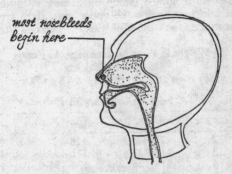

most nosebleeds begin here

FIGURE 22. *Usual site of nosebleed.*

Bleeding from high in the nose will gush out both nostrils and fill the throat. No pressure of fingers will arrest this bloody torrent; nor will ice packs, pressure on the back of the neck, or other folklore remedies. Nasal hemorrhage flowing from both nostrils calls for urgent medical attention; rush to the doctor or the nearest hospital emergency room.

Recurrent nosebleeds may signal underlying disease. In youngsters, the cause may be an allergy that provokes chronic nasal congestion, although rarely a case of leukemia or Hodgkin's disease will be found. In adults, high blood pressure, cancer of the nasal membrances, or blood disorder may announce its presence by recurrent nosebleeds.

OBESITY

Synonym: overweight

One of every three Americans is overweight, and obesity is the leading cause of preventable disease in America. Diabetes, atherosclerosis, heart disease, and scores of other ailments are adversely influenced by obesity.

Are you overweight? The scales tell the story and doctors sometimes put a number value on obesity by measuring the skin fold thickness behind the upper arm. Here are tables of desirable weights for various heights for men and women:

Weight in Pounds According to Frame
(in Indoor Clothing)
for Men and Women Aged 25 and Over

Height—Men (Shoes with 1″ heels)

Feet	Inches	Small Frame	Medium Frame	Large Frame
5	2	112–120	118–129	126–141
5	3	115–123	121–133	129–144
5	4	118–126	124–136	132–148
5	5	121–129	127–139	135–152
5	6	124–133	130–143	138–156
5	7	128–137	134–147	142–161
5	8	132–141	138–152	147–166
5	9	136–145	142–156	151–170
5	10	140–150	146–160	155–174
5	11	144–154	150–165	159–179
6	0	148–158	154–170	164–184
6	1	152–162	158–175	168–189
6	2	156–167	162–180	173–194
6	3	160–171	167–185	178–199
6	4	164–175	172–190	182–204

Height—Women (Shoes with 2″ heels)

Feet	Inches	Small Frame	Medium Frame	Large Frame
4	10	92–98	96–107	104–119
4	11	94–101	98–110	106–122
5	0	96–104	101–113	109–125
5	1	99–107	104–116	112–128
5	2	102–110	107–119	115–131
5	3	105–113	110–122	118–134
5	4	108–116	113–126	121–138
5	5	111–119	116–130	125–142
5	6	114–123	120–135	129–146
5	7	118–127	124–139	133–150
5	8	122–131	128–143	137–154
5	9	126–135	132–147	141–158
5	10	130–140	136–151	145–163
5	11	134–144	140–155	149–168
6	0	138–148	144–159	153–173

For girls between 18 and 25, subtract one pound for each year under 25. (Courtesy of Metropolitan Life Insurance Company)

A quick calculation of your ideal weight is as follows: For both men and women, allow one hundred pounds for the first five feet of height, then add five pounds for each additional inch in women, six pounds in men. Thus a 66-inch-tall woman should weigh 130 pounds. For large frame, add an extra 10 percent.

Perhaps the most personalized estimation of your best weight is the weight at which you felt trim and attractive in your twenties.

Calories count, and despite the extravagant claims of authors who promise that you'll lose pounds and inches on their 14-day eat-all-you-want magic diets, long-term weight control demands attention to calories, including the energy released by the metabolism of foods and calories burned per hour of activity.

Attacking Obesity

Obesity can be overcome, but it will take diligence and sacrifice.

First some calculations are in order. From your present weight, subtract your calculated ideal weight. Let's say that the difference is 20 pounds. That means that you have to shed 20 pounds to fit into your new bikini bathing suit or your ten-year-old tuxedo.

Next, calculate the number of weeks you wish to spend losing the weight. A weight loss of one pound a week is leisurely, two pounds weekly is a little ambitious. If you plan to lose one pound a week, it will take five months to shed the 20 pounds.

Then begin keeping a diet diary, writing down everything put into your mouth and calculating the calories per serving using the calorie guide found in the appendix of this book. By the day's end, you will probably find that you have eaten 2,500 calories or more. If coupled with a somewhat sedentary life, such a high-calorie diet is likely to add weight around the hips and middle.

Next calculate what must be eliminated from the diet. A key figure is this: Each pound of weight equals 3,500 calories. Thus, to lose one pound a week, 500 calories daily must be eliminated from the diet. That sounds easy: cut two slices of white bread and a large piece of cake (or the equivalent) from each day's intake, and you will lose one pound a week if all other factors remain stable. To lose two pounds weekly, 1,000 calories must be eliminated from each day's menu.

Once the diet is begun, continue writing down each bit of food, including indiscretions. I advise patients to eat their food early in the day, and if following a 1,200-calorie diet, they should take about 400 calories each meal. Those counting calories strictly soon discover that high-carbohydrate treats and fatty foods cost too many calories, and they are most satisfied with a diet high in protein, high-fiber vegetables, and fruits.

Burning up Calories

We should pay attention not only to calories consumed, but to their end use. Calories consumed must be burned or they will be stored as fat, and any diet calculation must consider the activity of the dieter.

Here's a list of approximate caloric values for daily activities. From this it's possible to calculate your caloric need each day. Figure approximately how many minutes you spend each day in vigorous exercise, sedentary activity, and sleeping.

- Strenuous activity burns 300 to 800 calories per hour: running, swimming, skiing, and heavy physical labor.
- Vigorous activity burns 200 to 300 calories per hour: golfing, cycling, riding, dancing, and heavy housework.
- Moderate activity burns 100 to 200 calories per hour: gardening, walking, and ordinary housework.
- Light activity burns 50 to 100 calories per hour: office work, cooking, and light housework.
- Sedentary activity burns 10 to 50 calories per hour: reading, eating, sitting, and sleeping.

When devising your ideal diet, remember that an increase in physical activity (be honest in your calculations) can help as much as eliminating the equivalent number of calories from the diet. A self-help home conditioning program is illustrated on page 39.

Getting Started

Today is a good day to start your weight control and exercise program. Motivation helps; if there's a picture of you that shows every bulge, tape it to the refrigerator door. Or perhaps buy a new bathing suit or gown to fit your ideal weight and size, then paste the label and price on the kitchen wall. Sometimes it helps to have a buddy; you and your partner can compare diets, exercise, and weights each week. Weight Watchers and similar diet organizations utilize this group therapy, together with dietary supervision and planned exercise.

A visit to the doctor is a good idea. You will receive a thorough checkup to exclude disease, and the physican may give much-needed diet guidance. Follow-up visits to his office help keep you on the straight-and-narrow path.

Sometimes the urge to snack is overwhelming, and the following foods, virtually calorie-free, make excellent emergency snacks:

Coffee and tea without milk or sugar
Sliced celery
Raw carrots
Bouillon
Pickles

Radishes
Lettuce
Gelatin dessert

It helps to begin each meal with a big glass of water or perhaps a cup of thin broth. Gravy, high-calorie salad dressing, bread and butter, rice, and potatoes are out. If hunger pangs are not assuaged, top the meal with a dish of low-calorie gelatin dessert.

A good book to buy and use is *The Low Calorie Diet* by Marvin Small (Simon and Schuster, New York) describing taste-tempting, calorie-pinching recipes such as eggs à la florentine (160 calories), asparagus milanaise (65 calories), and Norwegian jellied lamb chops (204 calories).

How about diet pills? Prescription diet pills are first and second cousins of the amphetamines, theoretically aiding weight reduction by reducing the appetite and perhaps increasing the metabolism. Unquestionably, much of their usefulness accrues from the placebo value of taking pills. If prescribed by the physician, well and good, but the prescription should not be refilled and these drugs should not be used without his supervision.

Available without prescription are several products said to reduce the appetite. The following may be helpful, although their placebo value probably overshadows any physical benefits:

- Di-Ette Reducing Plan contains methyl cellulose, caffeine, phenylpropanolamine, and vitamins.
- Slim-Mint Tablets contain methyl cellulose, dextrose, benzocaine, and flavoring. Silm-Mints are taken before meals to reduce appetite, or following meals as dessert.
- Melozets Wafers contain methyl cellulose with a wheat-flour base. When taken with water before meals, Melozets produce stomach-filling bulk.

Group therapy, ritual weighing, medical consultations, and weight reducing tablets may all help, but the secret of weight reduction is balancing calorie intake against energy output, not only during the period of active dieting, but for the rest of your life.

OSTEOMYELITIS

Synonym: bone infection

A bone infection may occur in any area, including the spine, leg, and even fingertips. The staphylococcus germ is the most common offender, and osteomyelitis may arise following an injury or bloodstream infection, although sometimes the cause is obscure.

Osteomyelitis causes bone pain and destruction, and eventually there may be drainage to the surface.

The treatment includes antibiotics and surgery, and long-term therapy is the rule.

OSTEOPOROSIS

Synonym: softening of the bones

Osteoporosis is a consequence of aging—the softening of bones that occurs due to low hormone levels and perhaps a poor intake of calcium and phosphorus. In the aging male and the postmenopausal female, body-building sex hormones are in short supply, and one of the many organs affected is bone. Calcium and phosphorus are lost, causing "thinning" of the bones, and fractures occur more easily than in younger individuals.

Osteoporosis may result in shortened stature as body weight compresses the spine, and buckling of the front portion of the vertebrae may cause a round-shouldered "dowager's hump." In time, arthritis may intervene, with persistent pain in the back and other joints.

What to Do about Osteoporosis

Diet can help. Needed are lots of protein and plenty of calcium and phosophorus. Lean meat is the best protein source, while milk (skimmed milk if you are wary of calories and milk fats) can provide bone-building minerals.

Pay attention to posture. Promote good posture habits by performing this exercise four times daily: Stand with your heels, hips, shoulders, and head against the wall. How good it feels to stand totally erect! Now slowly inhale, and release, two full breaths, then walk across the room with your head held high as though trying to brush the ceiling with your hair.

Practice walking tall whenever possible, and don't slouch in chairs. Good posture habits can help avoid a round-backed look in old age.

The doctor may prescribe hormones—estrogens for women, and sometimes anabolic (body-building) or androgenic hormones for men. Their advantages are weighed against their dangers, and your physician is your best source of advice concerning their use.

PALPITATION

Synonyms: skipped beats of the heart, pounding in the chest

Palpitation describes an awareness of the heart's action, which may be described as a rapid or irregular heartbeat, pounding in the chest, or a vague fluttering of the heart. In some individuals, palpitation is constant, while other persons describe intermittent episodes, perhaps during times of anxiety. Some victims report palpitations only during stressful situations, while others are awakened from sleep with an ominous sensation of cardiac malfunction.

Coping with Palpitation

Self-help therapy can often overcome heart palpitation. Sometimes a rapid or irregular heartbeat is caused by the stimulant action of coffee or tea, and elimination of caffeine-containing beverages will prevent palpitation. In other individuals, smoking plays a role, and cessation of tobacco use may bring relief.

When palpitation is traced to anxiety, it helps to lessen the responsibilities of everyday life: avoid overtime work, shun evening meetings, resign from committees, and postpone new projects.

Natural remedies include traditional sedatives such as lettuce, cabbage, or camomile with honey. Here's one recipe: Add three ounces of lettuce and one-half ounce of camomile to one quart of water and cook for 30 minutes to make lettuce leaf-camomile broth; drink one cup of the broth with breakfast and supper.

PARKINSONISM

Synonym: paralysis agitans

Parkinsonism, a neurological disease named for Dr. James Parkinson, who first described the illness more than 150 years ago, is a disease of middle and old age that causes a tremor of the hands and impaired walking, with difficulty initiating movement and a tendency to lurch forward or backward. This gait is hesitant, with small steps, and the body often bends forward from the waist during ambulation. The facial expression appears fixed and masklike and the patient often suffers emotional lability (instability) with depression.

Parkinsonism is caused by damage to tiny nerve cells of the brain, called basal ganglia, and may be related to an infection such as viral encephalitis or to arteriosclerosis. In addition, certain drugs, including phenothiazine tranquilizers, can cause symptoms of paralysis agitans.

Treatment

Parkinsonism calls for patience and understanding on the part of other family members. When the victim of paralysis agitans speaks, the speech may be muffled or slurred, or there may be hesitation and stuttering. Resist the urge to supply the "right word"; let the patient finish his sentence. Depression is common, but cheery settings and a hopeful word can help lift a dark mood. Life should be made as easy as is practicable for the parkinson patient: the toilet should be handy to the bedroom, climbing stairs should be minimized, and the patient should be spared tasks requiring complex digital dexterity.

Exercise helps. A stroll each day keeps muscles limber; games that require the use of small muscles (such as checkers or dominoes) should be encouraged; and, whenever possible, allow the paralysis agitans victim the dignity of buttoning his own clothes, cutting his own food, and performing the complex small duties of daily living, even if it seems to take him hours to complete the task

Drug treatment of parkinsonism is making new strides each day. Don't be satisfied with yesterday's drug treatment when new medicines may bring relief. Following is a list of antiparkinsonism drugs that may help:

- Trihexyphenidyl hydrochloride (Artane) has long been a widely prescribed antiparkinsonism agent, reducing tremor in most individuals treated. Side effects may include dry mouth, drowsiness, mental changes, and others. The usual starting dose is 1 mg, increased to a usual dose of 6 to 10 mg daily.
- Procyclidine hydrochloride (Kemadrin) and biperiden hydrochloride (Akineton hydrochloride) are chemically related to trihexyphenidyl and have similar actions and side effects.
- Benztropine mesylate (Cogentin) has a long duration of action and is often taken at bedtime. Its usefulness against the tremor and rigidity of parkinsonism must be balanced against its frequent side effects, which include dry mouth, sedation, and mental changes.
- Levodopa (Dopar, Larodopa, L-dopa) has come into general use during the past ten years. Scientific studies show that levodopa brings improvement in at least 50 percent of patients if the drug is given for six months or more. Side effects may include nausea and vomiting, dizziness, mental changes, involuntary movements, and more. Side effects are reduced if the drug is taken as Sinemet, combining levodopa with carbidopa, which boosts blood levels by delaying the metabolic breakdown of levodopa.
- Amantadine hydrochloride (Symmetrel) is the newest drug to receive approval for the treatment of paralysis agitans. Symmetrel was introduced several years ago to protect individuals exposed to certain types of viral flu. Since then its beneficial effect on parkinsonism has been proven, and studies have shown that patients who respond to amantadine will also usually have a favorable result following levodopa treatment.

Brochures describing the management of paralysis agitans and detailing helpful exercises are available. Write to:

PEPTIC ULCER

Synonyms: stomach ulcer, gastric ulcer, duodenal ulcer

A peptic ulcer is the price many persons pay for the hectic pace of life in the 1970s. Responsibilities piled upon obligations lead to late hours, short tempers, and monumental frustration. As emotions boil, peptic juices are produced by the bucketful, eroding the lining of the stomach and duodenum.

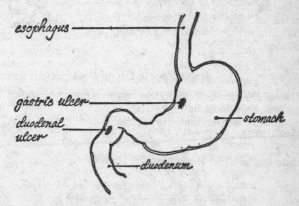

FIGURE 23. *Site of gastric and duodenal ulcers.*

Most ulcers form in the duodenum—the first part of the small intestine—as stomach acid nibbles away at delicate cells lining the intestinal wall. Less common are ulcers in the stomach, called gastric ulcers (See Figure 23). The gastric ulcer worries the physician, since an apparent ulceration may later prove to be cancerous, but malignant change in a duodenal ulcer is as rare as an honest politician.

Both duodenal and gastric ulcers produce identical symptoms—heartburn in the upper abdomen and lower chest, worst after meals and particularly aggravated by coffee, alcohol, and spicy food. The severe burning subsides somewhat after drinking milk or taking antacids, only to return later. Noctural pain is common, as excessive acid causes burning when the stomach is devoid of food.

Long-standing and poorly treated ulcers often lead to complications. Bleeding is common, sometimes occurring in the absence of pain, and is manifested as dark, black bowel movements, with progressive weakness as blood is lost into the stomach and intestines. Perforation of the stomach or duodenal lining may occur in a deep-seated ulcer, causing excruciating abdominal pain, while long-standing ulcers may cause scar tissue that obstructs the flow of food.

Treatment

During the acute phase of ulcer symptoms, therapy includes an ulcer diet, with bland creamed foods and milk taken often to neutralize stomach acid as soon as it is formed.

ˊAcute Peptic Ulcer Diet

General Diet Rules: No food to be eaten except as shown below. Feedings must be taken regularly as listed. Milk should be at room temperature. No alcoholic drinks, tea, coffee, or aspirin.

Acute Peptic Ulcer Diet—General Diet Rules:

8 A.M. — One portion of cooked Farina, Wheatena, or Cream of Wheat with sugar and one-half glass of cream. One slice of toasted white bread with butter. One glass of milk.

10 A.M. — One glass of milk.

12 noon — One portion of creamed soup with strained vegetables, such as celery, mushrooms, or asparagus. Mashed, baked, or boiled potato with butter. Plain Jello, or cornstarch, custard, rice, or tapioca pudding.

2 P.M. — One glass of milk.

4 P.M. — One glass of milk.

6 P.M. — One cup of creamed soup with vegetables. Mashed

baked, or boiled potato with butter. One portion of poached egg. One glass of milk.

8 P.M. — One glass of milk.

Bedtime — One glass of eggnog, malted milk, buttermilk, or half-and-half.

Antacids, such as Riopan, Gelusil, or Maalox, are often taken to aid in neutralizing stomach acid. One or two teaspoonfuls (check the directions on the bottles of these over-the-counter medications) may be taken every two hours during the day and upon awakening at night. All antacids are sold over the counter; do not buy antacids by prescription since the pharmacist will add his professional fee for handling a prescription.

When ulcer symptoms are severe, the doctor will usually prescribe an anticholinergic medication to suppress acid formation. Common choices are propanthelene (Pro-Banthine), glycopyrrolate (Rubinul), or dicyclomine hydrochloride (Benty). One tablet or capsule is usually taken three or four times daily and sometimes the doctor will advise a double dose at bedtime. Side effects include dry mouth and constipation, although a slight dryness of oral secretions is considered a useful sign that the drug is working.

When peptic ulcer symptoms are severe, rest is needed. Emotional tension should be at a minimum, and responsibilities must be put aside for a while. In addition, the doctor will often prescribe a mild tranquilizer such as oxazepam (Serax), diazepam (Valium), or meprobamate (Equanil). Available without prescription are the antihistamine "sedatives" such as Compoz.

Once acute ulcer symptoms have subsided, dietary restrictions can be relaxed, and the patient graduates to a chronic ulcer diet. Although more liberal than the initial list, the chronic ulcer diet follows the basic principles of taking frequent feedings of bland foods, with plenty of milk to neutralize stomach acid.

Take an eight-ounce glass of milk between meals and at bedtime.

Foods Permitted	Foods to Be Avoided

Cereals

Cooked oat and wheat cereals	Sugar-coated cereals
Dry precooked cereals	
Bran cereals	

Breads

White bread	Whole wheat bread
Muffins, rolls, and biscuits	Pancakes and waffles
Corn bread	

Soups

Creamed soups	Bean, lentil, or split pea soups
	Bouillon and broth

Meat, Fish, and Dairy Products

Boiled, baked, or broiled veal, ham, lean beef, turkey or chicken, and fish	Mutton and pork
	Fried or fatty meats
	Shellfish
Soft cooked eggs	Fried eggs
Cheese	
Cottage cheese	

Vegetables

Cooked or pureed vegetables	Raw vegetables
Carrots	Cucumbers
Lettuce	Brussells sprouts
Peas	Onions
Potatoes	Turnips
Spinach	Radishes
Corn	Tomatoes
Cabbage	
Beets	
Celery	
Asparagus	
Green beans	
Squash	

Fruits

Cooked or pureed fruits	All raw fruits
Dilute fruit juices	Apples
Bananas	Pineapple
Apricots	Grapefruit
Dates	

Foods Permitted	Foods to Be Avoided
Pears	
Prunes	
Oranges	
Melons	
Plums	
Peaches	
Figs	
Raisins	

Desserts

Foods Permitted	Foods to Be Avoided
Custard and pudding	Cakes
Ice cream	Pies and pastries
Sherbet	
Gelatin	
Tapioca pudding	
Cornstarch, rice, or bread pudding	

Beverages

Foods Permitted	Foods to Be Avoided
Cocoa, Postum, and Ovaltine	Coffee, tea, and alcohol
Milk	Decaffeinated coffee
Skimmed milk	Carbonated beverages
Buttermilk	

Miscellaneous

Foods Permitted	Foods to Be Avoided
Liquid vegetable oils (corn, soybean, and safflower)	Animal fats and lard
Nuts	Pepper
Macaroni and spaghetti	Olives
Garlic	Pickles
Jelly and jam	Tomato paste
Honey and molasses	Mustard
	Horseradish
	Relish
	Vinegar

After several months have passed without symptoms, and perhaps after an upper-gastrointestinal x-ray has revealed healing of the ulcer, medication can often be discontinued and most dietary prohibitions lifted. But be wary. The ulcer tendency remains, and the individual who has suffered a peptic ulcer must be forever wary of aspirin and other ulcer-irritating drugs, of coffee and alcohol, and of prolonged periods of emotional stress. Medication should be kept at home, and the diet list carefully saved. At the first sign of ulcer symptoms, recurring, begin strict adherence to the ulcer diet, start taking the medication (be sure you've asked the doctor or pharmacist if the prescription is refillable), and call the doctor as soon as possible.

PERIARTERITIS NODOSA

Synonym: polyarteritis nodosa
Periarteritis nodosa is one of the collagen diseases, so called because these disorders involve the collagen (connective cells of blood vessels, muscles, and other supporting fibers of other body tissues).

Polyarteritis nodosa causes fever, often linked with asthma and a skin rash.

Sometimes the cause is traced to a medication—possibly penicillin, sulfa, iodine, or anticonvulsant drugs. Treatment of this rare disorder may include cortisone, plus elimination of any suspected cause.

PERITONSILLAR ABSCESS

Synonym: quinsy
A deep abscess in the area of a tonsil has long been known as quinsy; it differs from an ordinary sore throat in that a distinct pus pocket is present. The patient complains of severe sore throat, fever is noted, and examination of the throat reveals severe swelling of one side, as shown in Figure 24.

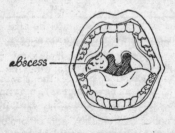

FIGURE 24. *Right peritonsillar abscess.*

Treatment

Warm salt water gargles help reduce swelling and relieve inflammation, but these merely supplement therapy prescribed by the physician. A throat culture will be taken to determine if a streptococcal infection is present, and antibiotics are usually prescribed.

As with other abscesses, cure demands draining the pus pocket. Often this occurs spontaneously, with the sudden discharge of a teaspoonful or more of pus into the mouth and throat. Pus and blood from the abscess should be spit out, followed by warm salt water gargles to aid healing. Sometimes the physician will elect to incise and drain the abscess using a scalpel and local anesthesia.

Once a peritonsillar abscess has occurred, most physicians recommend that the tonsils be removed to prevent recurrence.

PINWORMS

Synonyms: seatworms, enterobiasis

Pinworms often infest school children, who acquire the eggs from playground dirt, school toilets, and other sites of contamination. Anal or even vaginal itching is common, both during the day and while sleeping. Mothers make the diagnosis by examining the rectum while spreading the buttocks wide apart, a maneuver best performed in the early morning as the child first awakens. Pinworms are seen as tiny silver threads, scurrying in and out of the anal opening.

The doctor can clinch the diagnosis by examining a sample taken by pressing Scotch Tape against the anal opening. Under the microscope he will see the pinworm eggs.

Eliminating Pinworms

The doctor will prescribe one of the standard pinworm remedies, such as piperazine (Antepar), pyrvinium pamoate (Povan), or thiabendazole (Mintezol). Usually the doctor recommends that the drug be taken by all household members.

Medication is only the beginning. To eradicate pinworms

from the household and prevent reinfection, the following steps should be taken:

- Youngsters' fingernails should be cut short and scrubbed several times daily.
- Scrupulous cleanliness and frequent hand washing must be the rule, so that pinworm eggs are not passed from hand to foot to mouth.
- All underwear, pajamas, and bedclothes should be boiled, then ironed.
- For two weeks following the onset of treatment, the towel and linen of the pinworm victim should be kept separate from those of other family members, then boiled again.
- The kitchen and bathroom should be cleaned with a good disinfectant (such as Lysol) to eliminate lingering pinworm eggs.

PITCHER'S ELBOW

Synonyms: Little League pitcher's elbow, epicondylitis

After seven innings, Johnny's elbow begins to hurt. He's been throwing curve balls again, in spite of the coach's instruction to avoid curves.

Johnny suffers epicondylitis, an inflammation of the elbow attachment of muscles that flex the wrist. The cause is repetitive motion, and most victims trace their symptoms to a throwing motion.

Pitcher's elbow is the "flip-side" of tennis elbow (*q.v.*). Pitcher's elbow strikes the medial epicondyle of the elbow while tennis elbow—due to extension at the wrist—affects the lateral epicondyle.

Treatment of Johnny's pitcher's elbow parallels that of tennis elbow: rest is enforced, and his throwing motions are forbidden. Moist heat is applied for 30 to 60 minutes four times daily. Aspirin may help relieve pain and inflammation, and occasionally the physician will inject the local area with cortisone.

PITYRIASIS ROSEA

Another of the skin diseases of obscure origin is pityriasis rosea, most often afflicting young individuals, more common in women than in men, and occurring most often during the spring and fall of the year. Pityriasis rosea affects the skin of the chest, neck, and upper arms, beginning with a "mother (or herald) patch" that is red, "branny" to touch, and perhaps itches slightly. A few days later many other patches develop; these resemble the mother patch but are smaller, oval, and parallel the ribs (see Figure 25).

No treatment is really needed; the eruption will disappear spontaneously within four to six weeks, and rarely returns. Itching can be controlled by the local application of diphenhydramine (Benadryl) cream, or the physician may prescribe an antihistamine tablet such as tripelennamine (Pyribenzamine) to be taken three times daily.

The disease is more worrisome than serious, and must be differentiated from psoriasis, syphilis, and fungus infections (*qq.v.*).

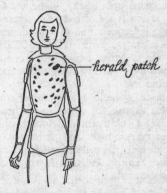

herald patch

FIGURE 25. *Pityriasis rosea.*

PNEUMONIA

Synonym: pneumonitis

Cough, fever, and blood-tinged sputum characterize pneumonia. Malaise is usually severe, and there may be shortness of breath. Rarely does pneumonia arise spontaneously. Rather, it usually follows a throat infection, common cold, or bronchitis, particularly in the very old, very young, or chronically ill. A fulminating lung infection is often the final episode in a series of debilitating diseases.

Dealing with Pneumonia

Some pneumonias can be prevented, Avoiding tobacco smoke helps prevent bronchial irritation that might make a fertile site for bacterial growth. Prompt and aggressive treatment of upper respiratory disorders, including strep throat infections, helps avoid a complicating pneumonia. Visitors with colds should be kept from the sickroom of an ailing patient.

When pneumonia is suspected, the doctor will make a definite diagnosis based upon x-ray, blood tests, and sputum examinations. Various types of bacteria, viruses, and even fungi may cause lung infections, and therapy depends upon identification of the causative germ. If bacteria are discovered, the doctor will often prescribe penicillin or one of its substitutes, depending upon the results of tests to determine bacterial sensitivity to antibiotics.

In addition to specific antimicrobial treatment, rest is prescribed, plus aspirin for fever; expectorants, such as glyceryl guaiacolate (Robitussin), to loosen phlegm; codeine to suppress unnecessary cough; and perhaps oxygen if shortness of breath is present. Convalescence is often prolonged, but most otherwise healthy individuals respond to appropriate treatment of pneumonia.

POISONING

Each year more than one million Americans suffer accidental (or occasionally deliberate) poisoning with household products or medication, and more than 2,000 of these victims fail to survive the toxic episode. Accidental ingestion of home medicines and other substances cause most childhood poisoning, while attempted suicide is the most common cause in adults.

Many times the so-called poisoning is inconsequential—a youngster tasted a drop of mother's perfume, chewed the end of a cigarette, or ingested a half dozen baby vitamins. But other times, poisoning can endanger life, and an understanding of certain principles can prevent mishaps.

The following five rules can help avoid accidental poisoning with household products:

- Keep all medicines and potentially toxic household products out of the reach of toddlers. There should be secure locks on the medicine cabinet and on the closet containing liquid bleach, hydrocarbons such as turpentine, and other potentially poisonous chemicals.
- Never tell a child that medicine is "candy." He may believe the ruse and hunt out the "candy" when hungry later.
- Keep all medication, especially flavored children's aspirin, in child-proof containers. And remember that these hard-to-open containers serve a useful purpose; replace the cap properly, don't leave it ajar.
- Laundry bleaching agents look like milk, and if left in a glass atop the washing machine may be grabbed and gulped by a thirsty toddler. Keep all potentially corrosive chemicals out of the reach of youngsters.
- Teach youngsters to respect the poisonous potential of medicines and household chemicals.

Treating Acute Poisoning

Each poisoning episode is an experiment in pharmacology. In all but the most minor episodes, a health-care professional should be consulted. A good source of advice is your nearest

Poison Control Center. There are some 580 poison control and information centers recognized by health officials; the following is a list of leading centers in each area of the United States:

New England

Poison Center
Children's Hospital Medical Center
300 Longwood Avenue
Boston, Massachusetts 02115
Telephone: (617) 232-2120

Vermont Poison Center
Medical Center Hospital of Vermont
Burlington, Vermont 05401
Telephone: (802) 656-2439

Middle Atlantic

Western New York Poison Center
Children's Hospital
219 Bryant Street
Buffalo, New York 14222
Telephone: (716) 878-7000

Poison Control Center
455 First Avenue
New York, New York 10016
Telephone: (212) 340-4494

Pittsburgh Poison Center
Children's Hospital of Pittsburgh
125 De Soto Street
Pittsburgh, Pennsylvania 15215
Telephone: (412) 681-6669

South

Poison Information Center
Children's Hospital
1601 Sixth Avenue South
Birmingham, Alabama 35233
Telephone: (205) 933-4050

Maryland Poison Information Center
University of Maryland at Baltimore
School of Pharmacy
636 West Lombard Street
Baltimore, Maryland 21201
Telephone: (301) 528-7701

Duke University Poison Control Center
Duke University Hospital
Durham, North Carolina 27710
Telephone: (919) 684-8111

Huntington Poison Center
St. Mary's Hospital
2900 First Avenue
Huntington, West Virginia 25701
Telephone: (304) 696-2224

Midwest

Poison Control Center
Children's Hospital of Michigan
3901 Beaubien Boulevard
Detroit, Michigan 48201
Telephone: (313) 494-5711

Poison Information Center
Academy of Medicine of Cleveland
10525 Carnegie Avenue
Cleveland, Ohio 44106
Telephone: (216) 231-4455

Milwaukee Poison Center
Milwaukee Children's Hospital
1700 West Wisconsin Avenue
Milwaukee, Wisconsin 53233
Telephone: (414) 344-7100

Southwest

New Mexico Poison and Drug Information Center
Bernalillo County Medical Center
2211 Lomas Boulevard, N.E.

Albuquerque, New Mexico 87106
Telephone: (505) 843-2551

Poison Center
University of Texas Medical Branch Hospitals
8th Street and Mechanic Street
Galveston, Texas 77550
Telephone: (713) 765-1420

Rocky Mountain

Rocky Mountain Poison Center
Denver General Hospital
West 8th Avenue and Cherokee Street
Denver, Colorado 80204
Telephone: (303) 893-7771

Intermountain Regional Poison Control Center
University of Utah Medical Center
50 North Medical Drive
Salt Lake City, Utah 84132
Telephone: (801) 581-2151

St. Louis Poison Center
Cardinal Glennon Memorial Hospital for Children
1465 South Grand Boulevard
St. Louis, Missouri 63104
Telephone: (314) 772-5200

Poison Information Center
Children's Memorial Hospital
44th Street and Dewey Avenue
Omaha, Nebraska 68104
Telephone: (402) 553-5400

Pacific

Fairbanks Poison Center
Fairbanks Memorial Hospital
1650 Cowles Street
Fairbanks, Alaska 99701
Telephone: (907) 452-8181

Thomas J. Fleming Memorial Poison
Information Center
Children's Hospital of Los Angeles
4650 Sunset Boulevard
Los Angeles, California 90027
Telephone: (206) 634-5252

Poison Information Center
Children's Orthopedic Hospital and Medical Center
4800 Sandpoint Way, N.E.
Seattle, Washington 98105
Telephone: (207) 634-5252

A finger down the throat may induce vomiting in the individual who is already suffering nausea due to the poison. Sometimes doctors recommend keeping syrup of ipecac in the home. Syrup of ipecac causes vomiting, usually occurring about twenty minutes after a 10 to 15 ml dose followed by a glass of water. Emptying the stomach better than lavage (stomach pump), ipecac-induced vomiting can remove toxic substances before absorption. A word of caution: *Never attempt to induce vomiting if the patient has taken a hydrocarbon, strong acid, strong alkali, or other corrosive substance.*

Sometimes useful is the universal antidote (Unidote), containing charcoal, magnesium oxide, and tannic acid. Unidote provides 15 gm of universal antidote in a four-ounce bottle. Immediately before use, fill the bottle with water and then drink the entire contents. However, note that the antidote has limited usefulness, and it should not be the sole therapy of potentially serious poisoning.

Ipecac may not always induce vomiting, and gastric lavage with a tube placed in the stomach avoids the long wait until a vomiting occurs, while reliably removing stomach contents. Requiring special equipment and training, stomach lavage is a job for the doctor.

Accidental poisoning is better prevented than treated, and constant vigilance concerning household chemicals is well worth the effort.

POISON IVY

Synonyms: ivy dermatitis, rhus dermatitis

Just as frigid winter weather is accompanied by colds and flu, warm summer days bring poison ivy dermatitis, afflicting millions of Americans each year. The cause is the resin of the poison ivy plant (genus Rhus or Toxicodendron), deposited on the skin while walking in the woods or acquired from the fur of an animal that has brushed against the plant.

A few days later the dermatitis appears—red, blistered, and itching intensely. The blisters may break to drain clear serum that, contrary to old wives' tales, will not spread poison ivy to other individuals.

Most commonly affected are the hands, wrists, neck, and face, although the resin may be transferred to cause lesions along the belt line, on the chest, or on the penis. Severe swelling may occur, particularly when the rash involves loose tissues around the eye, on the back of the hand, or on the penis.

Treatment

Self-help therapy may suffice in mild poison ivy dermatitis: weeping blisters should be dried by soaking with a warm Epsom salt (hydrated magnesium sulfate) solution—one teaspoonful of Epsom salt to one pint of warm water—applied as a moist compress for 30 minutes every four hours. When oozing is no longer present, itching can be assuaged by applications of Calamine lotion, Rhulicream, or by a poultice of grated raw potato.

Moderate to severe cases should be treated by the physician, who may administer cortisone by injection and/or pills, perhaps supplemented by antihistamine tablets for itching. A cortisone cream may relieve itching and speed healing, as may applications of the gel of the Aloe Vera plant.

Preventing Poison Ivy

Poison ivy is best prevented by avoidance. This means staying away from fields or woodlands known to be infested with the weed; climbing vines on trees are often poison ivy. Youngsters who have spent the day playing in the woods or fields should strip completely and shower thoroughly with a strong soap and lots of water.

Poison ivy injections help build resistance to the dermatitis and are sometimes recommended to individuals who suffer repeated episodes of severe rhus dermatitis. Widely used is Ivyol brand of poison ivy extract, administered in a dose of four injections the first year followed by a booster dose each spring.

POLIOMYELITIS

Synonyms: polio, infantile paralysis

Until a generation ago, polio was an ever-present threat of childhood. During the early twentieth century, epidemics were common, with summer camps closed and youngsters prohibited from swimming. Today the disease is rare indeed, thanks to the development of an effective vaccine.

Polio is caused by a virus that enters through the mouth and causes a minor illness resembling an intestinal virus with headache, nausea, vomiting, diarrhea, and fever. Most cases progress no further and subside leaving natural immunity. But in a few individuals the polio virus enters the brain and spinal cord, causing muscular aching and stiffness, often followed by a paralytic weakness in major muscle groups, and usually involving the extremities. In time, nerve deterioration is followed by muscle shrinkage, resulting in the shriveled limb characteristic of infantile paralysis.

Preventing Polio

Polio is preventable. The first breakthrough came in 1952 with the development of the Salk poliomyelitis injectable vaccine, superseded later by the Sabin trivalent live oral poliomyelitis vaccine. The live vaccine, given orally and mimicking the natural infection, induces excellent immunity, and the self-help attack on polio means keeping your vaccine up to date (see Immunizations).

For further information about polio write to:

The National Foundation—March of Dimes
P. O. Box 2000
White Plains, New York 10602

POSTNASAL DRIP

Synonyms: chronic postnasal discharge, phlegm in the throat

Millions of persons suffer chronic postnasal discharge, awakening in the morning gagging with mucus, clearing the throat and occasionally coughing during the day. Some individuals report a seasonal variation, while others note that their postnasal discharge continues unabated all year round.

Tobacco smoke, inhalants, allergy, and sinus infection may all contribute to postnasal discharge, and proper treatment follows discovery of the cause.

Alleviating Postnasal Drip

Smoking is a prime offender, irritating delicate membranes of the nose, sinuses, throat, larynx, and trachea. Cessation of tobacco use is the first step in effective therapy.

Inhalants other than tobacco smoke may play a role. These include automobile exhaust fumes, industrial pollution, household dust, insecticide sprays, and many others. Elimination of irritating inhalants may bring relief.

A common contributing cause is allergy, perhaps to the pollens of trees and weeds, to airborne molds, or house dust. Pollen allergy sufferers will report a seasonal variation, while the dust-allergic individual may find his symptoms most pronounced during winter months.

Symptoms may be relieved by the use of antihistamine-decongestant medication such as:

- Coricidin-D Tablets containing chlorpheniramine, phenylephrine, caffeine, and aspirin.
- Dristan Tablets containing phenindamine, phenylephrine, caffeine, aspirin, and an alkaline buffer.

Chronic severe symptoms may respond to allergy testing, followed by desensitization injections.

If sinus infection is present, one or two 30-mg nonprescription pseudoephedrine (Sudafed) tablets taken three times daily may bring relief. (It's noteworthy that 60-mg Sudafed Tablets require a prescription, while 30-mg Sudafed Tablets are sold over-the-counter.) The doctor may also prescribe an antibiotic such as penicillin or tetracycline (Achromycin-V).

Some persons report that postnasal drip disappears when they move to a warm, dry climate, but the symptoms of this minor disorder rarely necessitate such a move.

POSTURAL HYPOTENSION

Synonym: transient low blood pressure

Standing abruptly after lying in bed or sitting in a chair can cause a temporary drop in blood pressure, resulting in momentary lightheadedness and even fainting. The phenomenon occurs in individuals with low blood pressure, afflicts some persons with otherwise normal blood pressure, and may be seen in hypertensive patients taking the medication guanethidine (Ismelin). Hardening of the arteries often plays a role, and postural hypotension is most common in older individuals but may occur at any age. Viral infection, including flu, seems to predispose to episodes of postural hypotension.

Prevention

Rarely is medical therapy needed, and postural hypotension is best avoided by constant vigilance. Arise gradually from bed, first sitting for a few seconds, then stand slowly and stay near the bed for a short while lest dizziness occur. After sitting, particularly for a prolonged period of time, stand up cautiously and leave the safety of the chair only after you are sure that dizziness hasn't occurred. Be particularly wary of working in a stooped position, as when gardening, since standing abruptly following squatting or bending may cause symptoms.

Postural hypotension occurring during therapy for high blood pressure should be reported to the physician.

PROSTATIC ENLARGEMENT

Synonyms: prostatic hypertrophy, prostatism

In contrast to prostatitis, the enlarged prostate is a disease of older men. The prostate gland surrounds the urethra, which carries urine from the bladder, and enlargement of the gland can squeeze off the urinary flow (see Figure 26). When this happens, the patient complains of difficulty initiating the urinary stream, and the flow of urine occurs in a stop-and-start fashion. The patient may arise from bed several times each night to pass urine, and urination may be followed by a sensation that the bladder has not been completely emptied.

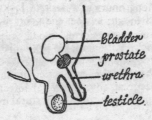

FIGURE 26. *The enlarged prostate gland can block urinary flow from the bladder.*

The doctor will confirm the enlargement of the prostate upon rectal examination, perhaps followed by cystoscopy—a look into the bladder using a tubular instrument (cystoscope) under anesthesia.

Although drug treatment has been attempted from time to time, there is no effective medical cure of the enlarged prostate. Surgery is the answer, and an operation will be advised when the enlarged prostate threatens to cut off the urinary stream or cause damage to the bladder.

PROSTATITIS

Synonyms: prostate infection, prostatosis

The male with prostatitis complains of frequent trips to the bathroom with a constant discomfort in the pelvis, perhaps radiating to the tip of the penis. There may be the urge to arise from bed at night to urinate, perhaps coupled with a burning upon passing urine. In contrast to an enlarged prostate, prostatitis is a disease of young and middle-aged men and, once present, shows a distressing tendency to recur.

Prostatitis begins with congestion of the prostate gland perhaps following inactivity such as riding in a car on a long trip or sitting for long hours at a desk. A lack of sexual relations seems to be a factor, as does the overuse of alcohol and coffee.

Sometimes infection is present, although other men suffer a noninfected engorgement of the prostate and some doctors call this condition prostatosis.

Relieving the Problem Prostate

An examination by the physician reveals the extent of the problem, and the doctor may massage the prostate to squeeze out a few drops of secretions that he can examine under the microscope. If infection is present, an antibiotic will be prescribed.

Periodic prostatic massage is an old-fashioned yet still effective treatment for prostatic congestion. The physician inserts a gloved finger in the rectum, and presses on the prostate to force out fluid causing congestion. Relief may last a few days or longer, and repeated massages may be required before the condition can be pronounced cured.

A self-help method of prostatic massage has been described: Lie on your back on the floor and flex both knees so that the feet meet sole to sole. Then slowly extend both legs as far as possible, keeping the soles of the feet together. Repeat the maneuver ten times morning and night.

Self-help therapy strives to avoid precipitating causes and prevent recurrences. Alcohol and coffee are avoided, although the physician may allow a cup or two of decaffeinated coffee each day. Long automobile rides are shunned, and yet, if unavoidable, should be interrupted by an hourly rest-stop and exercise. By the same token, the desk-bound executive should rise every half hour or so, walk to the window, stroll down the hall, and learn to think on his feet.

Exercise helps relieve congestion, mobilizing body fluids into the circulation. A daily exercise period helps prevent prostatic congestion, and patients often report that they feel no symptoms when active, yet suffer the return of discomfort when sitting watching television. Useful activities include mowing the lawn, walking the dog, painting the fence—virtually anything to get the patient on his feet and moving about.

Unless specifically forbidden by the doctor because of acute infection, sexual relations help empty the prostate gland. As one patient comments, "It's a lot more fun than a prostatic massage."

A natural remedy for prostatic congestion is eating squash seeds, said to aid the normal function of the prostate gland.

Following a course of therapy, the prostatitis victim may be symptom-free for months or years, only to note the gradual return of urinary frequency and prostatic discomfort—perhaps following an ill-advised long motor trip and/or the overuse of alcohol. When symptoms recur, prompt therapy is needed; begin the self-help measures described and see the doctor promptly.

PRURITIS ANI

Synonym: rectal itching

Itching about the rectum is a most distressing symptom that can pose a worthy challenge to both self-help care and medical science. Sleep is interrupted, and during the day there is the overwhelming urge to scratch. Elimination of the itching depends upon accurate diagnosis and prompt therapy. Here are some causes and cures:

- Fungus infections often invade the area near the rectum, a warm moist area that favors the growth of germs of all types. Over-the-counter treatment with tolnaftate (Tinactin) cream applied locally three times daily often brings relief if the diagnosis is correct, and the therapy should be continued for at least one week after all symptoms have ceased. Candidiasis (moniliasis) is a special type of fungus infection discussed in detail on page 64. Frequently involving the rectal and genital areas, candidiasis requires prescription treatment—often Mycostatin brand of nystatin cream applied three or four times daily.

- Chafing, sometimes called sweat dermatitis, is another cause of itching of the anal-genital area, often occurring in individuals who wear occlusive clothing such as nylon underwear, or who sit for long hours on leather or plastic seats, as well as in athletes who perspire profusely during exercise. A thorough daily shower should be followed by a dusting powder such as ZeaSORB, containing a corn cob derivative, or Johnson's Baby Powder containing talc. A ventilated seat cushion helps, and occlusive clothing should be discarded in favor of loosely fitting, well-ventilated, natural-fiber garments.

- Hemorrhoids cause anal itching, often associated with bleeding and a palpable lump. Hemorrhoid treatment, including the use of sitz baths, Tucks, and antihemorrhoidal ointments, is discussed on page 157.

- The anal fissure is a crack in the lining skin, typically caused by a large bowel movement that passes with the tissues incompletely relaxed. A stinging pain may be associated with the itching and a tiny streak of blood may be found on the feces. The local application of Rectal Medicone Ointment four times daily relieves symptoms and helps heal the fissure.

- Pinworms often announce their presence with rectal itching, sometimes most severe at night. For therapy, see Pinworms.

- Hypersensitivity reactions may occur near the rectum, often following the use of medicated creams and ointments. Common offenders are products containing mercury—neomycin, benzocaine, ethylenediamine stabilizers, and paraben preservatives in many prescription creams and ointments. A local contact rash may also follow the use of nickel clasps or pins on sanitary pads. The dermatitis subsides once use of the offending medicine or metal is stopped, and it is often best not to complicate a hypersensitivity dermatitis with other medication, although the doctor will sometimes prescribe betamethasone (Valisone) or similar cortisone cream to relieve symptoms.

- Medicine and foods taken by mouth can cause rectal itching. Spicy foods may be the culprit, as may a leaking oily laxative, but prime offenders are antibiotic tablets and capsules that may cause anal pruritis with or without candidiasis. Taking liberal amounts of buttermilk and yogurt can help avoid this complication of antibiotic therapy.

PSORIASIS

Psoriasis, a skin disorder of unknown cause, strikes five million Americans, and Richard B. Stoughton, M.D., Chief of Dermatology at the University of California, has written that "about 500,000 of these [individuals] have very serious difficulties finding anything resembling a normal life." The disease produces pale, silvery, scaling patches on the extensor surfaces of the body as shown in Figure 27. New areas of involvement often itch, but chronic long-standing patches are often pruritis-free. Individuals with advanced psoriasis may suffer multiple patches on the elbows, knees, back, chest, and scalp, perhaps associated with pitting of the nails and arthritis of the joints.

Fighting Psoriasis

The doctor has no cure for psoriasis, but can do much to combat the disease, and self-help methods augment his therapy.

A number of over-the-counter preparations are available, and these contain some of the same ingredients as prescription remedies (but cost less since there's no "prescription-handling" markup):

- Alphosyl Lotion, Cream, and Shampoo contain coal tar, a long-standing and useful psoriasis remedy. The cream and lotion also have soothing allantoin.
- Tar Doak Lotion contains 5 percent coal tar distillate plus mineral oil and lactic acid.

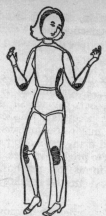

FIGURE 27. *Where psoriasis strikes.*

- Tegrin Cream and Shampoo, widely advertised, contain coal tar extract and allantoin.
- Siroil Emulsion contains mercuric oleate, mineral oil, and cresol.

These nonprescription remedies, when used according to package directions, can relieve the suffering of psoriasis. Local reactions are a danger, particularly if mercury derivatives are used. Change medications if a reaction develops.

Natural sunlight aids psoriasis, and a good summer tan can minimize skin involvement. During winter months ultraviolet light therapy, used at home according to the manufacturer's directions and the doctor's prescription, can replace summer sunshine.

Therapy beyond this point requires prescription medicine, and the doctor may advise the use of a cortisone cream, cortisone tablets or injections, ultraviolet light treatments, Vitamin A acid, or even the use of potent but somewhat dangerous methotrexate.

For more information plus some helpful treatment tips, write to:

National Psoriasis Foundation
6415 S.W. Canyon Court
Portland, Oregon 97221

PSYCHOSIS

The psychoses are the major forms of mental illness, comparable to neuroses as pneumonia is to a common cold. These disabling disorders pervade all aspects of mental function and sometimes necessitate long-term hospitalization, although the use of major tranquilizers during the past two decades has allowed many psychotic patients to leave mental hospitals and return to productive lives.

Three leading forms of psychosis are schizophrenia, paranoia, and manic-depressive psychosis.

Schizophrenia

Schizophrenia is the most common of the psychoses, usually beginning in young adults and accounting for the majority of admissions to mental hospitals. The old-fashioned term was dementia praecox, suggesting premature mental deterioration. It has been estimated that one in every hundred Americans will be treated for schizophrenia at some time during his life.

A wide variety of symptoms may occur. Early indications of schizophrenia may include an undue fascination with fantasy, a preoccupation with the mystical, an exalted attitude of self-importance, and an inability to relate to peers. The early schizophrenic is out of step with his family, his community, and himself. He marches to his own tune, and often retracts into a solitary existence.

In time he withdraws from the world about him and lives a fantasy existence. Some call him moody, others indifferent, and still others consider him odd or eccentric. If closely questioned, the disruption of his thought processes becomes apparent, and delusions, hallucinations, and loss of contact with reality may be exposed.

Paranoia

The individual with a paranoid psychosis suffers the twin delusions of believing that he has a sacred purpose and that others plot to thwart him. He may see himself as an avenging angel, as the last guardian of righteousness, or even as possessing a valued token or mystical object.

And no one else understands. If he hears whispers, they must be talking about him. Distant laughter is sure to be at his expense. Out there, somewhere, people are plotting against him. In desperation, he may commit violent acts—all "justified" in his mind. The individual who fires into a crowd on the street, and is later described by friends and family as "a good boy who worked hard in school," probably suffers a paranoid psychosis.

Manic-Depressive Psychosis

The manic-depressive psychotic has a cyclical personality with broad swings of mood. During depression he suffers a lack of pep and loss of interest in his surroundings. The appetite is poor, and sleep is interrupted by early morning awakening. He feels down in the dumps, may cry often, and suicide is a threat. Individuals with advanced disease may sit for hours without moving, lose weight, and fail to speak.

Then the mood swings, and the patient becomes elated, restless, and thoughts flow like machine-gun bullets. His self-confidence soars, and he may begin ten projects simultaneously, all doomed to failure as his interest shifts from hour to hour. As the manic stage progresses, all defenses crumble and mental processes may fuse into an uncontrollable delirious excitement.

Helping the Psychotic

The neurotic patient knows he's neurotic; not so with the psychotic, whose symptoms cause him little or no anxiety. The neurotic knows he is "not quite normal." The psychotic thinks he is normal, even especially gifted, and all about him are a little queer.

Thus the family and friends of the psychotic must take responsibility for guiding the patient to professional help. A visit to the doctor is the first step, and the family physician will recognize the presence of a severe mental derangement and arrange a referral to a psychiatrist, or perhaps a direct admission to a mental hospital.

The treatment of psychosis involves protection of the individual from self-harm; psychotherapy; and medication.

261

Protection from self-harm includes keeping the psychotic individual out of the hands of unscrupulous salesmen and exploiters who would profit by his lack of judgement. Severely depressed individuals must have dietary supervision, and the paranoid must be protected against his aggressive impulses.

Psychotherapy of the psychotic patient calls for the expertise of a trained psychiatrist. No lesser professional is qualified, and deep psychotherapy should not be undertaken by a family physician, clinical psychologist, religious adviser, or other professional unprepared to deal with the problems that may be uncovered. Psychotherapy often is initiated in the hospital, then continued on an out-patient basis following discharge.

Drug treatment has opened the doors of mental hospitals. The prototype of antipsychotic drugs is chlorpromazine (Thorazine)—invaluable in the treatment of schizophrenia. Related useful compounds include promazine (Sparine) and trifluoperazine (Stelazine).

If the patient is depressed, the prescription may be for amitriptyline (Elavil) or imipramine (Tofranil); lithium may be prescribed if the diagnosis is manic-depressive psychosis.

Once initial therapy has begun, family and friends of the psychotic patient can help by following these suggestions:

- Don't push the patient into new situations and social gatherings. Be patient and allow him to seek his own level of social activity.
- Avoid overprotections that seems to say: "You're still sick and can't be trusted."
- Allow him a few idiosyncrasies—seemingly pointless rituals, a skipped meal here or there, or an odd turn of phrase.
- Don't hesitate to discuss the hospital experience and current therapy with the patient, but don't pry if he seems to resent discussing his illness.
- Assume a positive attitude: an illness has been suffered, it's under treatment, and the outlook is optimistic.

Learn all you can about mental illness. One recommended book is *Supportive Care: Theory and Technique*, by Werner M. Mendel (Mara Books, Los Angeles), telling how therapist and family can help and support the individual with a chronic psychosis, especially schizophrenia. Educational material is available by writing to:

> The National Association for Mental Health, Inc.
> 10 Columbus Circle
> New York, New York 10019

Finally, urge the psychotic individual to keep in touch with his doctor. Perhaps only a monthly appointment is needed; or maybe he'll see the doctor only three or four times a year. But a regular checkup lets the doctor probe for emerging symptoms and can allow the early therapy that might prevent an acute flare-up of the psychosis.

Q-FEVER

Q-fever is an uncommon infection caused by a Rickettsia organism—a germ of the same family that brings typhus and Rocky Mountain spotted fever. Ticks sometimes spread the disease, which causes chills and fever, headache, cough, and muscular aches.

The sporadic case usually escapes diagnosis, since a viral flu is the apparant cause of symptoms. If you have reason to suspect Q-fever, ask the doctor to order a specific test for the disease.

The treatment of Q-fever is tetracycline or chloramphenicol, plus rest, fluids, aspirin, and lots of time.

Further information about Q-fever is available from:

> Department of Health, Education, and Welfare
> Public Health Service
> Center for Disease Control
> Atlanta, Georgia 30333

RESUSCITATION

The emergency techniques of maintaining breathing and heart action are called resuscitation. The need always arises suddenly, and may follow a heart attack, stroke, or automobile accident. The brain can survive only a few minutes in the absence of breathing and heartbeat, so prompt knowledgeable action is mandatory.

Mouth-to-Mouth Resuscitation

Mouth-to-mouth resuscitation is the recommended method of assisting respiration. Lay the patient supine on a coat or blanket and clear the airway by removing mucus, blood, or vomitus from the mouth with your finger, then open the air channel by arching the head back while grasping the lower jaw with your fingers beneath and thumb in the mouth to depress the tongue. Next, place your mouth over the patient's mouth: with children, your mouth will also cover the youngster's nose; with adults, block the nose by pinching the nostrils with your other hand. Breathe deeply, then exhale with moderate force into the patient's mouth, watching his chest rise, then fall. Repeat this maneuver 12 to 16 times each minute until normal breathing resumes or until care is given over to an ambulance attendant or physician.

Cardiac Resuscitation

When the heartbeat stops, cardiac resuscitation is needed. The approved method is closed heart cardiac massage, applying pressure to the breastbone that compresses the heart against the spine—rhythmically emptying, then filling the heart chambers. The patient must be lying flat on his back on a firm surface; if he is in bed, place a wide board, or even door, beneath his back or lift him to the floor. Standing or kneeling to the side, place one hand over the breastbone (sternum) and the other hand on top of the first. Then using your body weight with the arms extended, forcefully press the sternum toward the spine, then release. Gauge the force of your thrust by the patient's age and size; ribs can be fractured by this maneuver, particularly in older individuals with brittle bones, and a flailing broken rib end can puncture the lung. Closed-chest heart massage is continued at a rate of 60 beats per minute, until a normal pulse is felt, or medical help arrives.

Since resuscitation involves both heart and lung function, it is best performed by a team of two individuals. But you may be alone and, if so, just divide your efforts between mouth-to-mouth resuscitation and closed-chest heart massage. Here's how: Press the chest for five beats, then move to the mouth for one deep breath, continuing your dual resuscitation efforts until the patient is revived or you are relieved.

RHEUMATIC FEVER

Rheumatic fever is the consequence of inadequately treated streptococcal infection and is a generalized disease that involves the heart, joints, and other organs. The onset of rheumatic fever usually follows a streptococcal throat or skin infection and represents a reaction of the body to the strep infection. Early symptoms are joint pain and swelling, muscle spasm, skin eruption, and often nosebleed. The victim—usually a youngster approximately six to eight years of age—is frequently found to have a heart murmur and laboratory tests help clinch the diagnosis.

The active disease persists for weeks or months, then subsides spontaneously, but often leaves residual heart-valve damage.

Treatment

Bedrest is enforced as long as evidence of rheumatic fever persists, followed by very gradual rehabilitation and close observation for recurrence. The doctor may prescribe aspirin as specific therapy for rheumatic fever, and his directions should be followed explicitly. Penicillin or other antibiotics will be used if streptococcal infection lingers, and cortisone is sometimes prescribed for severe heart disease.

The outlook for the patient with acute rheumatic fever depends upon the extent of heart involvement. The individual who has suffered the disease must be protected against recurrences, with daily penicillin tablets or monthly penicillin injections recommended. Long-term follow-up is important in assessing the presence and extent of heart-valve damage.

In recent decades the incidence of rheumatic fever in America has declined drastically thanks to careful examination and treatment of possible strep throat infection in children, and prevention of this possible complication is

ample justification for seeking medical advice when a severe
sore throat is present.

ROSACEA

Synonym: acne rosacea

Usually striking adults rather than teen-agers, rosacea
causes a lively redness of the cheeks and nose. The rosacea
victim is sure to be accused of imbibing alcohol, and there
may be a grain of truth here, since rosacea is sometimes aggravated by alcohol as well as by coffee, tea, cola drinks, or
chocolate. Excessive skin oiliness is common, along with forehead acne and dandruff of the scalp.

Treatment

Self-help medical treatment of rosacea begins with dietary
restrictions. Alcohol, coffee, tea, cola drinks, and chocolate
are eliminated from the diet, as well as minimizing the intake
of greasy foods (French fries, potato chips, and other fried
foods) and refined carbohydrates (candy, sugar, and pastry).

Local therapy available without prescription is directed
toward removing excessive skin oils—without producing further inflammation. Choose the strongest soap that will get the
job done without irritation. Extra mild is hypoallergenic Purpose Soap, containing fatty acids and glycerin. For those requiring a stronger cleanser there is Seba-Nil Cleanser for Oily
Skin, containing acetone and polysorbate. Inflamed rosacea
sometimes responds best to Acne-Cort-Dome Lotion (prescription required).

If you consult the physician about rosacea, ask his opinion
concerning tetracycline treatment. This oft-prescribed antibiotic changes the composition of skin oils (accounting in part
for its beneficial effect on teen-age acne), and may be the
on-the-nose therapy for troublesome rosacea.

But when it's the night of the country club dance, or
you're speaking before the P.T.A. and want to look your best,
facial rosacea can be masked using Waterproof Covermark—
a cover-up cosmetic that blends with the normal complexion
to mask blemishes large and small.

ROSEOLA

Synonym: roseola infantum

Roseola is a virus infection of the "measles" family. Most victims are infants in the first year or two of life, and the disease follows a characteristic clinical course: high fever rages at 102°F to 104°F—up and down for about three days. Mother worries and the doctor ponders. Then, about the third day, the fever falls abruptly and a fleeting rash begins on the neck and face and spreads rapidly down the body, only to disappear at the end of a day or two.

That's all there is to the disease. Treatment consists of aspirin to control the raging fever, supplemented by sponging with tepid water when necessary. Fluids are given for dehydration and parents should keep a wary eye open for complications such as an ear infection or bronchitis (perhaps seen as a draining ear or intractable cough).

No vaccine is available and recurrences are rare. The doctor has nothing to add to self-help treatment, and neither he nor mother can diagnose roseola with certainty until the rash occurs.

RUBELLA

Synonym: German measles

German measles presents little threat to youngsters, who suffer only a low-grade fever, swollen lymph glands behind the ears, and a spotted rash that begins on the face and neck before spreading to cover the body. Symptoms last only a few days, and little therapy is needed other than rest and time.

Rubella poses its major threat to the pregnant woman. If German measles is contracted during the early months of pregnancy, miscarriage is common, and the fetus that survives until birth may suffer defects such as cataracts of the eyes, deafness, harelip, cleft palate, and congenital heart disease. Studies have shown that infected mothers will have miscarriage rate of about 10 percent, and another 20 percent will deliver infants with major congenital defects.

What to Do about Rubella?

Our best protection against rubella-damaged infants is elimination of the disease from society. This is done through "herd immunity"—the widespread use of vaccines so that epidemics are avoided and pregnant women aren't exposed. The live rubella-virus vaccine (Meruvax) should be given to all susceptible boys and girls from age one-year to puberty. Vaccination of postpubertal males is of low priority, but teen-age and adult women should be tested for immunity to rubella by the HI (hemagglutination inhibition) test. If the HI test shows immunity, vaccination is unnecessary. The postpubertal woman found to be susceptible to German measles may receive the vaccine if she understands that she must not become pregnant for the next three months and that some adult women suffer joint pains as the result of the live rubella-virus vaccine.

As with other live vaccines, the live rubella-virus vaccine should not be given to individuals who are pregnant; who suffer an acute febrile illness; who have leukemia or other blood disorders; who have a deficiency of gamma globulin; who are allergic to duck, chicken, or neomycin; or who are receiving treatment with cortisone, anticancer drugs, or radiation therapy.

The nonimmune woman exposed to German measles during the first three months of pregnancy may find herself at the center of a controversy. Today physicians often advise that the pregnancy be aborted; traditional management has been the injection of a dose of gamma globulin. If faced with this dilemma, be sure that all available tests have been done and rechecked, then seek the advice of a physician experienced in this field.

The Child with Rubella

This brings us back to the five-year-old child with a low-grade fever, rash, and swollen glands behind the ears. If there have been a few other rubella victims in the same kindergarten class and your child doesn't appear too ill, then the diagnosis seems reasonably certain and self-help treatment is fluids, rest, and aspirin for fever. A visit to the doctor will probably add nothing to your diagnosis and therapy; it might expose your child to another infection; and—perhaps most important—your child with rubella might infect an unsuspecting expectant mother in the doctor's waiting room.

SALMONELLOSIS

Synonyms: typhoid and paratyphoid fevers

Although uncommon in the United States, an occasional outbreak of typhoid or paratyphoid fevers occurs. Caused by bacteria of the salmonella family, these disorders produce fever, vomiting, diarrhea, abdominal pain, and prostration. Most individuals recover with or without treatment (although treatment markedly shortens the duration of symptoms), and an occasional victim, like the legendary Typhoid Mary, becomes a chronic carrier of the disease.

Prevention

Strict adherence to sensible rules of sanitation will prevent most infections. Only water from reliable sources should be consumed. If traveling in an area where the water supply is suspect, ask for bottled water in restaurants and insist that you personally open the cap (otherwise an enterprising waiter may refill empties with tap water). If bottled water is unavailable, boiling is the most reliable method of assuring pure water, although not always practical. Seasoned travelers tell me that two drops of tincture of iodine or Clorox in a tumbler of water kill most germs, as will five Halazone Tablets per quart (but wait 30 minutes before use). Be careful that harmful bacteria are not acquired during toothbrushing; in the hotel, let the water run 'til it's hot before rinsing the toothbrush. Tap water hot enough to be uncomfortable to the touch is unlikely to contain harmful bacteria.

Symptoms suggesting salmonellosis are evaluated by diagnostic tests, with blood and stool specimens submitted to the laboratory. If present, the disease is treated with chloramphenicol (Chloromycetin) or ampicillin (Polycillin).

Prophylaxis of salmonellosis includes typhoid vaccine, recommended for travelers to areas where sanitation is questionable.

If you want to learn more about salmonella infections, write to:

Center for Disease Control
Atlanta, Georgia 30333

SARCOIDOSIS

Synonym: Boeck's sarcoid

Sarcoidosis fits into no convenient pigeonhole. It seems not to be an infection, although sarcoidosis has been linked with tuberculosis. Lymph glands enlarge as in a malignancy, yet sarcoidosis does not follow the course of cancer. An allergic hypersensitivity may play a role, and there have been efforts to link the disease to pine-tree pollens.

More common in blacks than in whites, sarcoidosis causes enlargement of the lymph glands in the neck, underarms, and in the chest, sometimes associated with inflammation of the salivary glands or eyes. Shortness of breath may be present, but the patient is usually not acutely ill. Treatment may relieve symptoms, but probably does not alter the outcome of the disease, and most individuals recover spontaneously after a few years.

Treatment

No real therapy is needed unless symptoms are troublesome. The patient should eat a nutritious diet, perhaps supplemented by a multivitamin capsule. Fresh air and exercise are helpful, as in any chronic disease.

If enlarged lymph glands, particularly at the base of the lungs, compromise breathing or endanger vital chest structures, the doctor may prescribe cortisone. If so, gastric irritation may be avoided by following a bland diet, and taking an antacid "chaser" after the cortisone tablets. A low-salt diet is a good hedge against the fluid retention common with cortisone therapy. As with any course of cortisone treatment, the doctor's instructions must be followed explicitly, and "extra doses" should not be taken.

Regular medical checkups document the course of the disease and allow detection of complications, should such occur.

SCABIES

Scabies occurs from time to time in the United States, the parasite burrowing into the skin of the hands, wrists, underarms, buttocks, and genitalia to cause intense itching. Scratching soon leads to multiple discrete skin infections.

The recommended prescription therapy is gamma benzene hexachloride (Kwell) applied to all involved areas as directed by the physician, and there is no effective nonprescription medication currently available.

SCARLET FEVER

Synonym: scarlatina

Caused by group A beta hemolytic streptococci, scarlet fever is essentially a streptococcal sore throat accompanied by a rash. Symptoms begin with chills, fever, headache, and sore throat. There may be a foul odor (sometimes described as "mousey") to the breath and pus pockets noted on the tonsils. Within a day or two, the rash appears—multiple tiny red spots, most prominent on the torso, accompanied by a flushing of the cheeks with pallor around the mouth, a red tongue with enlarged papillae ("strawberry" tongue), and accentuation of the rash in skin folds of the underarm, elbow, groin, and neck.

If untreated, the fever and sore throat persist for five to six days, with the rash lasting longer and eventually scaling and peeling. Complications are common, including ear infection, pneumonia, and neck-gland infections. Rheumatic fever involving the heart and glomerulonephritis of the kidney may follow scarlet fever, as well as other streptococcal infections.

Treatment

The doctor will diagnose scarlet fever when he notes the typical sore throat, rash and fever, and his clinical impression will be confirmed by finding streptococci on a throat culture.

Scarlet fever responds promptly to penicillin—often given

by injection, followed by oral medication. Ten days of therapy are mandatory for all streptococcal infections, and a repeat throat culture should be taken at the end of treatment to assure success of therapy. Patients allergic to penicillin may receive erythromycin (Ilosone) or a similar antibiotic.

Self-help therapy supplements antimicrobial treatment. Aspirin is given for fever, and rest is advised until all symptoms have subsided. Warm salt-water gargles soothe the inflamed sore throat and fluids should be taken liberally. Dishes, utensils, towels, and other personal items used by the patient are considered contaminated, should be washed separately, and boiled if possible. The return to school should be deferred for at least one week, and probably until the repeat culture has confirmed the absence of all strep germs.

Household contacts should keep a watchful eye out for fever, sore throat, or rash—and the appearance of any of these requires a visit to the doctor and a throat culture.

SCHISTOSOMIASIS

Synonym: blood flukes

More than 150 million persons in the world are infected with the schistosoma blood fluke, which lives in snails and releases its larvae into water. Individuals bathing in this water acquire infection as the larvae enter through the skin and penetrate blood capillaries. From there, some schistosomes journey to the liver, others to the bladder.

Symptoms may be abdominal pain, diarrhea, and liver enlargement, or perhaps bloody urine.

Once the diagnosis has been confirmed, the physician may treat schistosomiasis with antimony potassium tartrate or stibophen (Fuadin).

The possibility of acquiring shcistosomiasis should be considered whenever a traveler is tempted to swim in tropical waters. Ask the local residents if the water contains snails and/or flukes. Infected areas include Brazil, Puerto Rico, Venezuela, Spain, Portugal, Greece, Africa, and many Oriental countries.

SCIATICA

Synonyms: slipped disc, herniated nucleus pulposus

Pain down one leg characterizes sciatica, an inflamation of the sciatic nerve composed of fibers originating in the spinal cord. The pain is described as aching or tingling, and numbness of the foot is often present. There may be weakness in extending the great toe, and often there is little or no perception of pin prick in the foot. In time, muscles of the leg may shrink, leading to permanent weakness of the extremity unless treatment is undertaken.

A slipped disc is the most common cause of sciatica. Problems begin when the cartilage disc between two vertebrae in the lower back slips into the spinal column, causing pressure on nerves exiting from the spinal cord. A backache is present, but it is often overshadowed by pain in the leg.

Treatment

Therapy is directed toward the lower back, the origin of the problem. Rest in bed for five to seven days usually helps, and local applications of heat may speed recovery. Good therapy is a long, hot tub bath, and hot, moist packs (perhaps using a Hydrocollator) are applied to the lumbosacral spine for 60 minutes four times daily. I often advise my patients to heat their Hydrocollator Pad in an electric stoneware cooker (crock pot) at the bedside.

Analgesics help relieve discomfort: aspirin may suffice, or the doctor may prescribe a stronger pain-killer such as propoxyphene (Darvon) or even codeine.

Sometimes the physician will order physical therapy treatments—ultrasound or diathermy. These provide heat to the deep areas, encouraging healing blood flow at the site of the problem.

X-rays should be taken, although ordinary back x-rays may look normal or may merely suggest the possibility of a slipped disc—described as "a narrowing of the interspace" between vertebrae. If a slipped disc seems to be the problem, the doctor will often perform a myelogram, an ex-ray examination of the spine, following the injection of a radioopaque dye into the spinal fluid.

If heat, rest, and medication lead to the relief of symptoms and disappearance of neurologic signs, well and good. However, persistent pain and neurologic deficits, if associated with a myelogram that suggests a slipped disc, are an indication for surgical removal of the slipped disc to relieve the symptoms of sciatica.

SENILITY

Synonym: senile brain disease

Chronic progressive hardening of the arteries impairs the blood flow to the brain and causes senility. Its course is variable, and no one knows why one individual "keeps his wits" until the ninth or tenth decade, while other oldsters seem a little "odd" in their late sixties or seventies.

An early symptom is forgetfulness—the victim has difficulty bringing a name to mind, hesitates in finding the right word, and loses personal items about the house. The individual with early senile brain disease may have difficulty remembering what he ate for breakfast or what he was told yesterday, yet often amazes friends and family by describing events that happened years before.

In time his forgetfulness may extend to personal habits, and he may neglect to shave or brush his teeth, and may even forget basic rules of politeness. Or on the other hand, some individuals become compulsively orderly, exhibiting fits of temper if their comb, brush, and personal cup aren't arranged "just so."

Mood swings may occur, and 'few changes may be noticeable over one or two decades, but the eventual picture is withdrawal as the mental factory gradually closes down.

Aiding the Oldster

Patience is the guide for coping with the somewhat senile older individual. When he fumbles for a word, resist the urge to fill the gap; rather allow him the dignity of completing his sentences. When he leaves articles around the house, their whereabouts sure to be forgotten, quietly return them to their proper spot, but suppress the urge to reprimand him.

The oldster's mood-swings must be borne with equanimity. When he's pleasant, enjoy it, but if Grandpa is in a grumpy mood, there's nothing to do but bear it; reacting with hostility threatens his security and may be met with an uncontrollable angry outburst.

The life of the senile individual must be simplified. Try to avoid presenting him with choices; alternatives are confusing. Be wary of changes; moving to a new home or even to a new room can cause confusion, particularly at night when his landmarks are lost. Whenever possible, medical treatment should be rendered at home rather than in the hospital. In a hospital the otherwise tractable older individual may become confused and obstreperous, and the nurses may react by shackling him to the bed, for fear that he may climb over the side and break a hip.

Darkness sometimes magnifies his disability and a night-light should be left on in the room and in the bathroom.

Steps can present a problem, and the oldster's bedroom should be on the same floor as his toilet.

Through it all, the dignity of the senior family member must be retained. Respect his advice, even though it is not followed, and honor his opinions even if you don't agree.

Sometimes the doctor can help by prescribing a vasodilator—a drug to open blood vessels to the brain. Papavarine (Pavabid) and nylidrin (Arlidin) are two examples. A glass of wine with meals may work just as well. The increased blood flow to the brain aids mental function in some, but not all, older individuals with cerebral arteriosclerosis.

Enlightened home care, perhaps aided by medication, can spell the difference between household harmony and discord, or perhaps between home care and institutionalization of a senior family member.

SHIGELLOSIS

Synonym: bacillary dysentery

Severe diarrhea with liquid stool that contains mucus and blood characterizes bacillary dysentery. Fever, vomiting, and abdominal cramps are present, and dehydration may result.

Bacillary dysentery is caused by Shigella bacteria, widespread in uncivilized areas of the world, and occasionally encountered in the United States.

Treatment

Fluid replacement is the major problem, and the patient should receive clear fluids, including water, Jello water, Kool-Aid, weak tea, and clear soups. Fluid losses via the bowel may be high and must be replaced by oral intake.

Over-the-counter Kaopectate may help reduce the frequency of bowel movements, but the physician should be consulted. He may prescribe camphorated tincture of opium (paregoric) or diphenoxylate with atropine (Lomotil) to curb diarrhea, as well as antibiotics such as ampicillin (Polycillin) to attack the Shigella infection.

The Shigella germs live almost exclusively in man, and prevention calls for good hygiene. Isolation of infected individuals is important, as is detection of the patient with mild shigellosis who may spread his disease to others unless treated.

SHINGLES

Synonym: herpes zoster

Shingles is one of the herpes infections, usually occurring as an elongated patch of blisters on the chest or abdomen (see Figure 28), but sometimes affecting the face or eye. The herpes zoster infection follows the path of a nerve, causing an intense deep pain, but limiting its infection to that part of the body served by the nerve. Initial symptoms of pain may precede the occurrence of blisters by several days, and herpes zoster infections of the right side of the abdomen have accounted for more than a few normal appendixes being removed.

The initial discomfort is soon followed by a crop of blisters, which break to form painful crusted sores. These persist for two to six weeks and then subside, although older individuals often complain of deep pain persisting long after the skin lesions have healed.

Herpes zoster infections involving the forehead place the

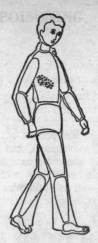

FIGURE 28. *Common site of shingles.*

eye in danger and demand a visit to an eye specialist. An early warning symptom may be a herpes blister near the tip of the nose, since the nerve fibers supplying the eye also serve this area.

Shingles, like cold sores, may come when the body's resistance is lowered by other disease, and shingles sufferers must be suspected of harboring other illness, possibly including cancer.

Recent medical evidence has linked the viruses of chicken pox and herpes zoster, and shingles may be considered the disease brought on in an individual who has partial immunity to the chicken pox virus.

What to Do about Shingles?

Because shingles are often linked to an underlying disorder, a search should be made for hidden infection, cancer, or other illness. If present, such disorder should be treated, so that the body's defenses are augmented.

The sores of shingles can be dried by careful us of an ultraviolet lamp, or the doctor may use the Spectroderm Lamp in his office. A good home remedy to dry oozing shingles blisters is compound tincture of benzoin, applied three times daily.

Cortisone is an effective remedy, and the physician may prescribe tablets or administer an injection, in hopes of preventing the persistent discomfort known as postherpetic neuralgia. Pain is a characteristic complaint, often responding to aspirin, but perhaps requiring a stronger analgesic such as propoxyphene (Darvon).

Herpes zoster infection of the eye, called herpes zoster ophthalmicus, requires skilled medical management, and often prescribed is an antiviral medication called idoxuridine (Stoxil).

SHOCK

Synonyms: hypotension, hypovolemia

Shock occurs with a sudden drop in blood pressure, seen as pallor, rapid pulse, impaired alertness, and a cold, clammy skin. The blood pressure may fall after extensive bleeding, as in a gastrointestinal hemorrhage due to bleeding peptic ulcer, or a blood loss following a severe injury. In other individuals the body's blood supply is intact, but blood pressure drops and circulation is impaired after a severe emotional experience, overwhelming bloodstream infection, or serious injury.

As with any life-threatening emergency, prompt knowledgeable treatment can be lifesaving.

Treatment

Shock therapy aims to restore blood to the vital organs in the central body core—heart, kidneys, liver, and lungs—and to the brain. First aid is as follows: Place a coat or blanket on the ground for insulation, then lay the patient supine. The legs should be elevated 12 to 18 inches, encouraging blood to return to the abdomen and chest by gravity. Then cover the victim with another coat or blanket for warmth. If he is fully conscious, small sips of water, tea, or warm coffee may be given, but not large quantities of liquids, nor should fluids be poured down the throat of a semiconscious shock victim.

Active bleeding is subdued by direct pressure with a clean handkerchief or scarf, holding firm pressure over the wound until all bleeding ceases or until relieved by an ambulance attendant.

Then, as soon as possible, the patient is transferred to a hospital. There the doctor will continue treatment, perhaps using intravenous fluids, including blood if bleeding has been severe.

The recovery rate following shock varies with the cause, but best results occur when first air is administered promptly and correctly, with professional follow-up as soon as possible.

SHOULDER PAIN

Synonyms: "bursitis" of the shoulder, tendinitis of the shoulder

Shoulder pain often follows vigorous physical activity, such as bowling, painting, and other sustained motion of the arm. Most such strains subside spontaneously, but occasionally acute inflammation develops, causing severe shoulder pain with inability to extend the arm to the side.

Although often called "bursitis" of the shoulder, the disorder is usually an inflammation of the tendon to the biceps muscle, properly called tendinitis. Little swelling is present, but there is tenderness to touch along the course of the biceps tendon at the front of the shoulder.

Even after therapy recurrences are common, and each flare-up deposits a small amount of calcium. Eventually a large calcium deposit may develop that acts as an irritant in the tissues.

Treatment

The painful shoulder may respond to self-help treatment. When acute pain upon motion is present, discomfort can be relieved by wearing a sling, but this is allowed for only a few days, since prolonged immobilization can lead to a frozen shoulder as tight scar tissue forms to impede motion of the joint.

Aspirin or Bufferin helps relieve discomfort and reduce inflammation; two tablets are taken with milk four times daily. Or the physician may prescribe a stronger pain-killer such as propoxyphene (Darvon).

Compresses can reduce inflammation and aid healing, although there is no general agreement whether cold or heat should be used. Some physicians insist that ice packs reduce swelling and are most effective, while other doctors claim that heat speeds healing by bringing blood to the inflamed area. I advise patients to begin with cold applications applied for 30 minutes every four hours; if relief is not attained with a day or two, heat should be used instead.

On about the third day, passive exercises should begin to restore normal motion to the shoulder joint. Begin by bending forward from the waist, moving the body so that the dangling arm rotates in an increasingly widening circle; repeat this exercise to a count of 20 four times daily.

Later come further passive exercises to increase range of motion (see Figure 29):

- Shoulder exercise 1: Sit on a chair beside the kitchen table with the arm stretched palm up across the table; then lean across the table, moving the trunk and neck so that the ear touches the extended arm.
- Shoulder exercise 2: Still sitting beside the table, extend the arm forward along the table, leaning forward until the shoulder touches the ear.
- Shoulder exercise 3: With the arm still resting on the table, flex the elbow; then bend forward from the waist, moving the nose toward the knees while leaving the arm on the table.

These exercises stretch shoulder ligaments to prevent scarring, without actively flexing the shoulder muscles. Passive shoulder exercises should be repeated four times daily until pain is gone and a full range of motion has been attained.

Severe shoulder pain should be treated by the physician, who may inject a combination of cortisone and lidocaine (Xylocaine), perhaps followed by physical therapy with ultrasound or diathermy.

Repeated episodes of bursitis or tendinitis with calcium build-up may require surgery.

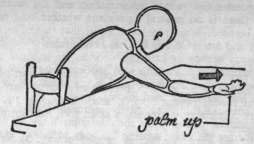

palm up

Shoulder exercise 1.

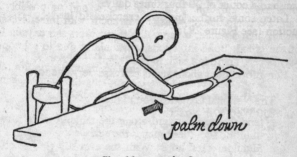

palm down

Shoulder exercise 2.

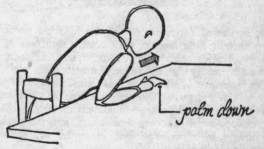

palm down

Shoulder exercise 3.

FIGURE 29. *Three exercises to increase motion of a stiff shoulder.*

SICKLE CELL DISEASE

The recessive gene for sickle cell disease is carried by 8 percent of blacks (and 0.5 percent of whites, particularly those of Mediterranean origin), and marriage of two sickle cell trait carriers may produce a child with full-blown sickle cell disease.

Sickle cell anemia, affecting one of every 500 black infants, leads to red blood cell clots within the arteries, causing impaired circulation, pain, skin ulcers, and/or possibly impaired consciousness. Attacks may occur with infection, anesthesia, high altitude, or anything that lowers the oxygen level of the blood. Bone infections, particularly due to salmonella, may occur. There is a high mortality rate.

For information about sickle cell disease, write to:

The National Genetics Foundation
250 West 57th Street
New York, New York 10019

SILICOSIS

Occupational exposure to silicon dioxide particles can cause chronic lung disease, with cough, shortness of breath, and progressive respiratory insufficiency. Silicosis victims have an especially high incidence of tuberculosis.

The treatment of silicosis is fresh air, exercise, expectorants such as glyceryl guaiacolate (Robitussin) to clear secretions from the chest, and perhaps inhalation therapy. Most important, occupational exposure must cease, and the patient cannot remain in an environment where he will inhale more silicon dioxide particles.

SILO FILLER'S DISEASE

Lung irritation due to nitrogen dioxide—formed when nitric oxide in fresh silage reacts with oxygen—causes silo filler's disease. The gas is formed when silage first comes in contact with air, and disappears within 10 days. An acute bronchitis develops when the nitrogen dioxide fumes are formed, and this accounts for the patient's symptoms.

Oxygen may aid impaired respirations, and the doctor should be called.

SINGER'S NODES

Synonyms: nodules of the larynx, vocal nodules

Small growths on the vocal cords may follow abuse of the voice—long hours of loud talking or singing—particularly if the voice is poorly pitched. Hoarseness and distortion of voice quality occur, worse after talking or singing for an hour or two.

Vocal nodules require rest of the voice. Talking is minimized, while shouting and singing are forbidden for a few weeks. Proper training may alter the pitch of the voice to minimize further formation of vocal nodules. Occasionally, persistent vocal nodules require surgery.

SINUSITIS

Synonyms: sinus trouble, sinus congestion.

Acute sinus infections cause facial pain, nasal stuffiness, and the achiness characteristic of infection. Nose blowing may result in a bloody discharge, and there may be headache and lassitude.

The common cold is a frequent precursor, and sinus infection begins as congestion blocks sinus openings, followed by the growth of bacteria.

Subduing Acute Sinusitis

The acute sinus infection usually responds to combination therapy, including decongestant medication, nasal drops or spray, warm facial compresses, and perhaps antibiotics.

Useful over-the-counter decongestants include 30-mg Sudafed tablets containing pseudoephedrine, or Dristan tablets containing phenylephrine and chlorpheniramine. Or the doctor may prescribe a more potent preparation such as dexbrompheniramine and d-isoephedrine (Drixoral).

Nasal drops and sprays open sinus channels, and a good choice is ¼-percent phenylephrine (Neo-Synephrine). More potent and also requiring no prescription is oxymetazoline (Afrin) nasal spray or drops, applied every 12 hours.

Warm moist compresses speed resolution of the sinusitis. Lie on the bed with a warm, wet washcloth across the nose and cheekbones, inhaling the warm vapor and allowing the heat to penetrate into sinus cavities.

Prescription antibiotics can eliminate bacterial infection, and the doctor will often advise the use of penicillin, erythromycin (Ilosone), or tetracycline (Achromycin-V) in a usual dose of one pill four times daily for five to seven days. Occasionally, a stubborn case of sinusitis requires surgical drainage by an ear, nose, and throat specialist.

SKIN CANCER

Three distinct types of skin cancers occur, each with its own distinct characteristics, recommended therapy, and outlook.

Squamous Cell Carcinoma

Squamous cell cancer of the skin can occur on any area, but is more common on those sites exposed to sunlight. A statistical study has shown that in the United States the incidence of skin cancer doubles every 265 miles, proceeding from north to south. Avoiding too much exposure to sunlight during youth and middle age can thus help to prevent skin cancer.

A rough, irregular, elevated growth that bleeds may be skin cancer, and all such lesions should be examined by the physician. Instead of debating whether it is cancer, he will usually excise the entire growth, along with a purdent margin of normal skin.

Basal Cell Carcinoma

Sometimes called the "rodent ulcer" because it burrows deep into normal tissues, the basal cell carcinoma is most often found on the face. Slow growth characterizes these tumors, which may bleed, then scab, then bleed again. Predisposing factors may include arsenic (Fowler's Solution), old burn scars, or skin exposure to tar and other hydrocarbons. Treatment may include surgical excision, electrosurgery, or perhaps x-ray therapy.

Malignant Melanoma

Arising from pigmented skin cells, the malignant melanoma is a more malicious neoplasm than the squamous or basal cell carcinoma. Some tumors grow out of a long-standing mole that undergoes change, while others arise from apparently normal skin. The usual appearance is a darkly pigmented area, less than half an inch wide, slightly raised from the skin surface, with irregular dark speckling. If you suspect the presence of such a growth, see the doctor, and *fast*. Malignant melanoma can kill, and early treatment is the only hope of cure.

If you're interested in learning more about skin and other cancers, read the Cancer section on page 60 and write to:

American Cancer Society
219 East 42nd Street
New York, New York 10017

SKIN SPOTS

Synonym: patches of hyperpigmentation

During middle age and later, large pigmented freckles may begin to develop. Most are found on exposed areas, their appearance influenced by past irradiation with sunlight. Those appearing on the face, hands, and shoulders present a cosmetic problem.

Bleaching Skin Spots

Lemon juice is an old-fashioned remedy, and sometimes works. Apply a small amount of lemon juice concentrate directly to the pigmented spots three times daily for several months. It may work, but stronger measures are often needed although there is no guarantee that they will be effective.

Two chemical products help bleach pigmented skin spots: hydroquinone and ammoniated mercury. Over-the-counter preparations containing these products include:

- Stillman's Freckle Cream containing ammoniated mercury and bismuth subnitrate.
- Ultra Nadinola Cream containing hydroquinone.

SNAKE BITE

Four types of snakes account for the approximately 3,000 poisonous snake bites suffered by Americans each year. Deaths are uncommon; the mortality rate for poisonous snake bites is about one percent, although survivors often suffer severe discomfort and local tissue damage.

The pit vipers, so-called because of a small depression between the nostril and eye, include the rattlesnake, copperhead, and water moccasin or cottonmouth. Several types of rattlesnakes are encountered, including the large diamondback, the prairie rattler, the timber rattler, and the small pigmy rattler. The bite of the copperhead, also called the Highland moccasin, is less dangerous than that of the rat-

286

tlesnake and is painful but rarely fatal. Riverbanks and swamps are the habitat of the water moccasin, which may, if disturbed, drop from a tree branch to inflict facial bites.

Pit vipers have fangs, and venom injected at the time of striking quickly causes local pain, swelling, and discoloration.

In a class by itself is the coral snake, whose bite causes multiple small fang marks (in contrast to the two distinct puncture wounds of the pit viper fangs). The coral snake bite causes little local reaction, but is soon followed by visual changes, slurred speech, and perhaps convulsions and death.

What to Do about Snake Bites

Caution can prevent many snake bites. Poisonous snakes attack in self-defense and bite when human beings disturb the reptiles unexpectedly. When walking in the woods, be wary of bright spots where snakes may be snoozing in the sun. Keep an ear peeled for the hollow, bony rattle that the rattlesnake shakes when disturbed. Wear thick leather, high-topped hiking boots, and look up as well as down when walking along a swampy riverbank.

But alas, you followed all the rules, yet a snake bite occurred. What to do?

First, identify the snake if possible. An accurate description of the reptile is helpful, but more positive identification is made by examination of the biting snake after it has been killed.

Lie quietly, since active movement speeds venom through the veins and lymph channels. Tie a tight tourniquet a few inches above the snake bite, then splint the extremity (one or two small tree limbs and adhesive tape or a magazine splint as shown in Figure 13, will do) to reduce motion of the extremity.

Check the tourniquet frequently; it should be just tight enough to wedge one finger beneath it, but should not block the arterial pulse.

Next scrub the wound with soap and water and apply whatever antiseptic is at hand; then make half-inch cross-shaped incisions through each fang mark and apply suction for at least one-half hour. Mouth suction is easily available, although a first-aid snake bite suction kit is preferable; old-timers describe using a heated jar or cup, the same technique used by doctors for "cupping" in the last century. In time, swelling may extend beyond the tourniquet, which should be moved centrally as swelling progresses.

After suction is discontinued, apply ice if available. This reduces pain and slows the action and spread of venom.

Finally, after the above first-aid measures have been completed, it's time to transport the patient to the doctor or hospital, moving slowly with splints restraining motion of the bite area.

The doctor will provide further local therapy of the snake bite, and will perhaps given an injection of polyvalent antisnakebite serum, as well as medication for pain and a tetanus booster injection if needed.

Poionous snake bites are but one of the many instances when proper emergency care can prevent pain and suffering, or even save a life.

SPINAL CURVATURE

Curvatures of the spine are found at any age, from young children to oldsters. They are classified in three general types according to the configuration of the vertebral column.

Scoliosis

Scoliosis is a lateral curvature of the spine, as shown in Figure 30. The cause is usually obscure and is often congenital. When mild, scoliosis causes no problem other than its cosmetic appearance, but severe scoliosis may hamper lung and heart function. An oft-neglected complication is shortening of one leg, and posture may be improved by adding a lift to one shoe.

Lordosis

Lordosis is the familiar swayback posture. Sometimes it is hereditary, and obese individuals may assume a swayback stance to balance a protruding paunch. Lordosis often responds to exercise that strengthen the spinal-supporting muscles, as described in Figure 7.

Kyphosis

Kyphosis describes a forward spinal curvature, including round shoulders, the familiar dowager's hump due to osteoporosis, or even the hump back. In days gone by, the hump back (or gibbus) was often caused by tuberculosis of the spinal column—called Potts' disease—typified by Quasimodo, the hunchback of Notre Dame.

A back brace to pull the shoulders into military posture

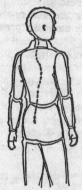

FIGURE 30. *Scoliosis of the spine.*

may help, and the kyphotic individual can help minimize his postural defect by conscientiously standing and sitting erect. Severe kyphosis, like marked scoliosis, can impair the function of the heart and lungs.

STOMATITIS

Synonym: inflamed mouth

Inflammation of the oral cavity is called stomatitis, coming from the Greek roots *stoma* meaning mouth and *itis* meaning inflammation. Pain is present and examination reveals red, irritated membranes involving the cheeks and gums, and perhaps the tongue. Proper treatment depends upon the cause of inflammation, whether dental decay, ill-fitting dentures, spicy foods, allergy, or viral infection.

Treatment

If present, dental caries must be corrected and poorly fitted dentures eliminated. Spicy dishes including hot peppers, pepperoni pizza, cinnamon, and highly seasoned foods are out.

Allergy sometimes plays a role, and a common offender is tooth paste or powder. Tobacco smoke may cause inflammation of oral tissues, and antibiotic use may cause local irritation as well as possibly leading to a yeast infection. Elimination of these irritants may speed recovery, and warm salt-water gargles four times daily will bring symptomatic relief. Carrot broth helps soothe and heal inflamed oral tissues, and can offer relief in nonspecific stomatitis. Use two ounces of carrot broth to rinse the mouth every two hours.

A suspected viral infection may also be treated with warm saline gargles, perhaps supplemented by a few drops of Gly-Oxide used to rinse the mouth following gargling.

Persistent stomatitis that resists all the above measures should be examined by the doctor.

STROKE

Synonym: cerebrovascular accident

Scientist Louis Pasteur, poet Walt Whitman, and actress Patricia Neal all suffered strokes.

Stroke, the third most common cause of death in America, trailing only heart disease and cancer, is a major cause of disability for many who survive the initial attack.

The stroke hits like a sledgehammer, felling active women and strong men. It may strike while sleeping, doing housework, or even in the middle of a sentence. Then, suddenly, speech is interrupted, an arm and leg are suddenly useless, one side of the face droops into a grotesque caricature, and there may be loss of consciousness. The doctor is called immediately and, unless the stroke is minor and already waning, he recommends hospitalization for medical treatment and physical therapy.

And so you may ask, "When faced with a disease that

strikes with alarming speed and apparent caprice, and that almost always requires professional care, what can the self-help practitioner do?"

Two things: first, many strokes can be prevented, as we'll see. And second, there is much that an interested family can do to aid the recovery of a stroke victim.

Preventing Strokes

The word stroke describes the loss of blood supply to a specific area of the brain. Sometimes there's a blood clot in a small artery, or there's bleeding (hemorrhage) within the brain cells. Whichever the cause, brain cells that have lost their blood supply fail to act, and those parts of the body that they govern lose their nerve control, become weakened, and cease to function—like an appliance without electricity.

The cerebral clot or hemorrhage occurs for a reason. Sometimes there's a weak spot in the artery, and this accounts for many strokes in younger individuals. In older patients, however, the cause is usually linked to hardening of the arteries, and stroke prevention is really avoidance of atherosclerosis. This means dietary diligence concerning cholesterol and fats, weight control, regular physical exercise, and all the other self-help tips described under Atherosclerosis.

Hypertension is often linked to strokes, and the cerebrovascular accident often follows soaring blood pressure levels—as bleeding breaks out at a weak spot in the vascular system. The individual with high blood pressure must take his medicine faithfully and check with the doctor regularly. The penalty for ignoring high blood pressure may be a sudden stroke.

Finally, major cerebrovascular accidents may be preceded by "small strokes"—transient episodes of slurred speech, weakness of a hand or leg, blurred vision, or other ill-defined neurological symptoms. If this happens, see the doctor promptly. He may find a sky-high lipid level, perhaps a bounding blood pressure, or other evidence that a major stroke is in the offing. And the physician may be able to avert the stroke by medication, rest, and dietary changes.

Stroke Rehabilitation

Recovering from a stroke means regaining speech, strengthening a weakened arm and leg, learning to walk again, and regaining dexterity in the hundreds of little chores we perform every day—cutting food on the plate, closing a zipper, and brushing the teeth. Physical therapy starts at the time of the stroke, progressing through the hospital stay and home care. The final goal is normal speech, full ambulation, and normal use of all extremities.

From the time of the initial stroke, medical and self-help care is aimed at eventual rehabilitation. Even while the patient is bedfast, there's much to do:

- A footboard at the end of the bed prevents foot-drop, with shortening of the calf muscles and Achilles' tendon. The footboard prevents bedclothes from forcing the toes down into a ballet position, and instead keeps the ankle square and toes pointed up in the air—a more physiologic position for eventual walking.
- A strategically placed pillow keeps a weakened leg from rolling to the side. Without support, the rotated leg may form scar tissue often requiring intensive therapy to overcome the tightness. The pillow (or sandbag) support keeps the toe of the bedfast patient pointed up and prevents the deformity.
- A rolled washcloth held in the weakened hand prevents a tight fishlike contraction following a stroke.
- Positioning a weakened arm in three different locations during the day helps to preserve full shoulder motion and prevent scar tissue formation. First, place the arm down along the side of the body with the hand near the hip; two hours later place the hand and forearm across the chest as though the arm were in a sling; then later, extend the shoulder so the arm is up along the head. Thoughtful arm and shoulder positioning early in the care of the stroke can avoid the need for painful stretching exercises later.
- As soon as the doctor gives his okay, start range-of-motion exercises to include all joints on the stroke side. This means that all the joints of the fingers, hand, wrist, elbow, shoulder, foot ankle, knee, and hip

are moved through their full range of motion, allowing several repetitions at each joint and repeated four times daily. For example, the wrist joint is flexed forward and extended back, bent to the right and then to the left, and then inverted from palm up to palm down—with each motion repeated two or three times. The same procedure is repeated for all other joints mentioned, being careful to get full extension at the knee joint, to extend the shoulder fully so that the upper arm lies along the head, and to preserve full motion in each of the small joints of the fingers and thumb.

Once the acute phase of the stroke subsides and the patient is out of danger, it's time to begin more active exercises, leading to use of a chair and then walking. Here are some helpful tips:

- An overhead trapeze helps the bed patient sit up, giving him a firm overhead support to pull against. Use of the overhead trapeze is also good exercise for the normal (and perhaps for the weakened) arm.
- Active exercises use the patient's own muscles. These, like the passive exercises described above, aim to reduce contractures and preserve range of motion, and they also help improve muscle strength and coordination. Top priority goes to moving joints through their full range of motion four times daily. If footdrop is a problem, a length of twine or string looped below the foot and held with both hands while lying in bed helps exercise the stiff ankle joint. A ball held in the hands, alternately squeezed and relaxed, builds hand and wrist strength.
- Start getting out of bed by having the patient sit on the edge of the bed for a few minutes three or four times daily. Once his balance is good and he feels ready to go, move to a chair. Anticipate dizziness the first time out of bed, and be ready to offer support under both arms. When the patient first stands, it's best to have the chair close at hand so he need only pivot and sit. The stroke patient will appreciate a not-too-soft chair with firm arm support. If the patient's strength and balance seem equivocal, use a chest re-

straint tied behind the chair as insurance. Since sitting in a chair is not as cozy as the warm bed, cover the knees and lower legs with a lap robe.

- Eating in a chair is more physiologic than consuming food lying in bed. And receiving a tray while sitting in a chair lends an air of accomplishment.
- Encourage the stroke victim to use the weakened hand; he must not be allowed to abandon it. Even though clumsy, he must use the hand for eating meals, buttoning clothes, and performing his daily toilet, as well as using the weakened leg to begin standing.
- Passing idle time with card games, dominoes, and puzzles helps improve small-muscle dexterity—if the patient uses the involved hand.
- When strength is sure and balance confident, it's time for walking to begin. In the hospital, parallel bars will be used first, perhaps followed by a walker or cane. At home, a walker is useful if there is good strength in the weakened arm. But when the stroke arm remains weak, it's often best to use a four-point cane held in the good hand. This means that all the weight goes on the good leg, and then, on the next step, half the weight goes on the stroke leg and half on the cane held in the opposite hand. Begin slowly. There's no rush. A few minutes is enough for the first day. Then gradually build up to four walking sessions daily— each one a little longer than the last if strength improves.
- Speech rehabilitation should begin with professional consultation. The speech therapist will diagnose the specific difficulty and start you on your way, perhaps with word and picture cards to build a basic vocabulary. Self-help speech therapy encourages conversation with the patient, particularly using those words and phrases suggested by the therapist.

Stroke rehabilitation can be one of the most rewarding of home-help nursing endeavors. Of course it takes patience. Results come slowly, and the home therapist will have to learn new procedures and skills. The following may be helpful:

- *Strokes: How They Occur and What Can Be Done about Them* by Page, Millikan, Wright, Weiss, Crawford, DeBakey, and Rusk, published in 1961 by Dutton; the advice remains timely—particularly Dr. Rusk's illustrated Chapter 8 discussing rehabilitation following a stroke.
- Send forty cents to the Superintendent of Documents, Washington, D.C., 20005, and request *Publication No. 596*—a useful pamphlet describing home care of the stroke patient.
- For information concerning a nearby rehabilitation service, contact the Association of Rehabilitation Centers, 828 Davis Street, Evanston, Illinois, 60201.
- And for timely advice concerning care of the stroke patient—including how to cope with bedpans, catheters, enemas, and the endless list of other chores that are part of home nursing—read *Feeling Alive after 65* by Robert B. Taylor, M.D., published by Arlington House, New Rochelle, New York.

The stroke victim needs and deserves first-rate medical advice and top-notch nursing care. But even more important, he needs cheerful surroundings, confidence in the care he is receiving, reassurance that everything possible is being done to hasten his recovery, and hope that he will become a productive family member once again.

STUTTERING AND STAMMERING

Stuttering-stammering is usually an emotional disorder. It begins as normal childhood speech hesitancy becomes magnified by parental overreaction and by the child's fear of failure. As such, stuttering is a type of performance anxiety, somewhat akin to stage fright, conversation hysteria, or even psychogenic impotence.

If the defect persists into adulthood, psychological problems can develop and the speech impediment may hamper the individual's job performance and his life.

Treatment

Family members must exercise restraint, suppressing the urge to supply the needed word. The youngster who shows signs of stammering needs reassurance by the parent that he can take his time forming sentences, that youngsters aren't expected to speak as fluently as adults, that he is loved no matter how he speaks, and—most important—that *there is nothing wrong with him.*

Of course therapy may be needed eventually, and if stuttering or stammering persist until the first or second grade in school, it is well for the child to have special speech training. Parents should still emphasize that the youngster is not sick but is taking an extra class in school to develop his skills in communication. If the school offers no speech therapy, a private practitioner should be consulted.

The adult with speech hesitancy should confront his problems squarely. Practicing speech before a mirror helps, as does reading aloud from a book or discoursing spontaneously upon an arbitrary topic. Some sufferers find improvement joining a public-speaking class, or perhaps a toastmaster's group.

If you or your youngster suffer stuttering or stammering, request information from:

National Association of Hearing and Speech Agencies
919 18th Street, N.W.
Washington, D.C. 20006

STY

A bacterial infection of an eyelash hair follicle is called a sty. A pus pocket forms and points to the surface, usually draining to discharge pus. There is slight local discomfort, and the eyeball may be red and irritated.

Treatment

Warm moist applications help subdue the infection, and should be applied for 30 minutes four times daily. The sty usually drains spontaneously, and should not be squeezed with the fingernails.

Sometimes the physician will prescribe an antibiotic eye ointment such as Bacitracin Ophthalmic Ointment to be applied four times daily following soaking, and occasionally antibiotic tablets or capsules are recommended. Recurrent sties may necessitate prolonged therapy.

SUNBURN

Injudicious exposure to sunlight can burn the epidermis as surely as hot water, causing a red, inflamed skin, often blistered, tender to the touch, and intensely painful. It seems that some individuals must, each summer, relearn the fact that sunlight burns unprotected skin.

Preventing Sunburn

The danger of sunburn is greatest between noon and four P.M., when the burning rays are strongest. Since sand and water reflect the sun's rays like a mirror, the danger of sunburn is greatest at the beach, somewhat less at poolside, and least while sunbathing in a grassy area.

Tanning lotions filter sun's rays and minimize the danger of burning. They may be washed away by sweating, and should be reapplied after swimming. Good choices include:

- Revlon's Sun Bath Moisturizing Tanning Lotion.
- Hypoallergenic Almay Deep Tanning Cream.

For maximum protection, a sunscreen is used. This product screens out most, if not all, of the sun's rays and is recommended for skin that seems to tan even through clothing and for those individuals who wish to preserve a fair complexion. Useful sunscreens are:

- A-Fil Cream containing titanium dioxide and methyl anthranilate.
- PreSun containing para-aminobenzoic acid.

Treating Sunburn

When sunburn occurs, self-help treatment includes cool compresses containing a tablespoonful or two of rubbing alcohol per quart. As the compresses are warmed by body heat and become dry, they should be remoistened. After the compresses are removed, allow the skin to dry without rubbing. Then apply a moisturizing cream. A good choice is After-Tan, containing a derivative of the Aloe Vera plant; some persons prefer direct application of the gel of the Aloe Vera plant.

In severe cases the doctor may prescribe the application of Aristocort-A Cortisone Cream, plus advice to avoid exposure to sunlight for the next few weeks.

SYPHILIS

Synonyms: lues, the "great pox"

Syphilis, caused by a corkscrew-shaped germ (spirochete) called Treponema pallidum, is usually passed during sexual contact, but can be acquired from individuals with open skin lesions, during transfusion, and can be passed from mother to child.

After an incubation period of about three weeks, the first evidence of syphilitic infection is seen as a chancre—a firm, elevated papule (pusless pimple) usually found on the penis or lips of the vagina. During this stage, the blood test for syphilis is negative or "doubtful," but examination of material taken from the chancre may show spirochetes under a darkfield microscope examination. Even if no treatment is received, the chancre subsides spontaneously, giving a false sense of security.

A "second incubation period" of 6 to 12 weeks precedes the secondary stage of syphilis. A skin eruption is common, often accompanied by sore throat, headache, fever, and lassitude. Sores may appear in the mouth; these are called mucous patches and abound in infectious spirochete germs. During the secondary stage of syphilis, the blood test is usually positive. After several weeks, the secondary changes of syphilis also subside.

Next comes a quiescent period of three to five years or more following the primary and secondary stages. During this time, called the latent stage, the blood serologic test for syphilis is positive.

Late syphilis may involve the skin, heart, brain, or other organs. Untreated late syphilis can cause severe mental changes, progressive heart disease, and sometimes death.

What You Can Do about Syphilis

Treatment of syphilis should, of course, be directed by the physician. Self-help advice concerns preventing syphilitic infection and recognizing the disease if and when it has developed.

Keep in mind the following facts about syphilis:

- Syphilis infections are on the rise. With the sexual revolution has come a sharp increase in the incidence of venereal infections, notably gonorrhea and syphilis.
- Syphilis respects no social barriers, and can be acquired from a "nice" girl or boy as well as from a more notably promiscuous sexual partner.
- Don't be fooled by a negative serologic test for syphilis drawn a few days after a worrisome sexual encounter. The blood test for syphilis usually doesn't become positive until two to four weeks after infection.
- Gonorrhea and syphilis can both be acquired from the same partner at the same sexual union. Yet the treatment for gonorrhea won't necessarily wipe out the spirochetes, and the gonorrhea victim should insist upon a blood test for syphilis three to four weeks after receiving antigonorrhea treatment.
- Although syphilis, like gonorrhea, must be reported to public health authorities, the heavy-handed official investigation is now usually a relic of the past. Most venereal disease case workers are sensitive to the patient's anxieties and conduct their findings in a discreet, low-key fashion.

For centuries, doctors have called syphilis "the great imitator," because its skin and internal manifestations can mimic dozens of other diseases. If you are concerned about a symptom and syphilis is a possibility, be sure to see the doctor and discuss your problem frankly. Don't hesitate to ask for a test for syphilis; it can sometimes be the key to a difficult diagnosis.

To learn more about specific social programs in the field of venereal disease, write to:

American Social Health Association
1740 Broadway
New York, New York 10019

TAY-SACHS DISEASE

Tay-Sachs disease is a genetic disorder affecting chiefly the descendants of Ashkenazic (German and Eastern European) Jews. This disease of infants and children causes blindness, mental retardation, and death.

Current emphasis is upon detection of genetic carriers of the Tay-Sachs recessive trait, with antenatal diagnosis (by analysis of fluid and cells from the pregnant uterus) followed by selective abortion of affected fetuses. A mass Tay-Sachs program of this type is currently in progress in the Washington-Baltimore area.

For further information, write to:

National Genetics Foundation
250 West 57th Street
New York, New York 10019

Tay-Sachs and Allied Disease Association
122 East 42nd Street
New York, New York 10017

TEETHING

The eruption of the first baby tooth is a milestone in an infant's life, and he announces the appearance of dentition with vocal acclamation. Fitfulness, crying, and poor feeding are common, and although many pediatricians disagree, mothers insist that there is an increased incidence of colds and viral infections while infants are teething.

Relieving Teething

The symptoms of teething are largely due to pain. Aspirin helps, and an average dose is one grain of baby aspirin per year of age taken every six to eight hours if necessary. That means that a seven or eight-month infant would receive one-half of a 1.25 grain baby aspirin tablet two or three times daily.

Teething rings filled with frozen fluid have been used for generations. My two children never accepted them, but the application of cold to the gums may be of some help.

Somewhat more effective are topical anesthetics applied to the gums. Most of these contain benzocaine and one widely available preparation is Benzodent. Topical anesthetics can be used every hour or two for relief of discomfrot, mindful of the possibility of sensitizing the infant to the drug, possibly producing an allergic reaction when that medication is used in later years.

Probably the greatest danger of ascribing fever to teething is the likelihood that more serious illness will be overlooked. Whether teething or not, youngsters with persistent high fever should be examined by the doctor, who will check for possible pharyngitis, ear infection, or other illness.

TENNIS ELBOW

Synonym: epicondylitis

Epicondylitis, an inflammation of a muscular attachment to the lateral elbow bone, occurs after many activities other than tennis. The common denominator is a forceful upward extension of the wrist and forearm, tensing the forearm muscles and tugging on their attachment at the elbow. I have treated patients with epicondylitis related to holding a heavy chain saw, wielding a hammer, using an overhead laundry press, and even holding a show-dog's head erect with pressure on a leash at an exhibition.

Pain is a constant symptom, and there may be tenderness with slight swelling near the lateral bone of the elbow (see

Figure 31). Symptoms are worse following activity that moves the wrist and forearm.

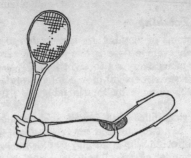

FIGURE 31. *Site of pain in tennis elbow*

Treatment

Therapy begins by eliminating the causative activity. Put the tennis racket away for a few weeks, or leave hammering to carpenters. Rest is essential if treatment is to be successful.

Heat aids healing; apply warm moist compresses for 30 to 60 minutes four times daily.

Aspirin helps relieve inflammation, but sometimes stronger medication is needed and the physician will often inject a combination of cortisone and lidocaine (Xylocaine). Surgery is rarely indicated.

If tennis-playing is the cause, using the two-hand backhand swing helps prevent epicondylitis.

TETANUS

Synonym: lockjaw

With each childhood laceration, my mother warned, "Wash that cut and apply some iodine or you'll get lockjaw." Several gallons of iodine and twenty years later, I learned in medical school that the fabled lockjaw of my youth was tetanus and that local care of minor wounds really does help.

Tetanus begins when the tiny Clostridium tetani germ enters the body via a puncture wound or deep laceration. Once inside, a toxin is formed that causes severe muscular spasm, including tightening of the jaw muscles (lockjaw). Spasm of the chest muscles prevents breathing, and tetanus infections may end in death.

Eluding the Tetanus Bacillus

Tetanus is a preventable disease. The vaccine against tetanus, called tetanus toxoid, affords remarkably good protection, and each case of tetanus that occurs today marks a failure of preventive medicine.

Tetanus toxoid immunizations begin at two months of age as part of the DPT injection (see Immunizations), and should be reinforced with a booster shot at intervals throughout life. "How often should I have a tetanus shot?" I'm often asked.

Older children and adults should have a routine tetanus booster every 5 to 10 years, unless one has been given to treat an injury. If a tetanus-prone injury occurs (a barnyard injury, a deep puncture wound, or a severe laceration), a tetanus booster is indicated if one has not been given during the last year or two.

If a tetanus-prone wound has been received and the patient has no knowledge of prior tetanus immunizations, the doctor may give tetanus immune globulin in addition to the usual tetanus shot.

Prompt and thorough local care of injuries helps prevent tetanus. ("You were right, Mom.") The tetanus germ likes dark, cozy places, so diligent scrubbing of wounds to clean dirt and potential infection from hidden recesses can thwart the tetanus bacillus.

Parents are often faced with the decision: should the doctor be called about a minor cut? Understanding the nature of tetanus helps guide the decision. Keep in mind that the tetanus germ lives in the intestinal tract of animals and enters the soil with animal droppings. The much-feared rusty nail injury is tetanus-prone, not because of rust, but because this outdoor menace may have acquired a tetanus germ from animal droppings and because its sharp point could inject that germ deep beneath the skin. I know of a tetanus infection that developed following a minor cut while slicing sausage; sausage casing is made from the intestinal tract of animals.

Therefore, medical care with a tetanus booster is recommended for individuals who have not had a tetanus shot for a year or two and who suffer:

- A deep puncture wound, particularly if acquired outdoors.
- A laceration that happens in the stable or barnyard.
- A deep laceration, such as in an auto accident.
- Any deep abrasion or laceration that is especially dirty.
- An injury with a knife or slicer that may have been used to cut sausage, pepperoni, or other byproduct of animal intestines.

THROAT INFECTION

Synonyms: sore throat, pharyngitis

Few of us escape the winter months without one or more throat infections. Children suffer more episodes than adults, probably owing to school-room exposure, a disinclination to wear appropriate outer garments, and lesser quantities of antibodies than adults who have weathered past throat infections.

First comes a scratchiness of the throat, followed by discomfort and difficulty swallowing. Fever may be present, as may be swollen glands in the neck and perhaps a cough. There is fatigue, loss of appetite, and occasional stomach cramps or vomiting.

Therapy of throat infections would be easy were it not for the specter of streptococcal infections. About one-quarter of all throat infections are caused by streptococci. In general, strep throat victims have sorer throats, higher fevers, and more tender swollen glands, but this generalization has many exceptions. It's important that strep infections be identified and treated aggressively because up to one percent of untreated streptococcal throat infections may result in rheumatic fever (perhaps leading to permanent heart damage) or glomerulonephritis (causing kidney damage).

Neither patient nor doctor can identify the strep throat infection without a throat culture, and thus a trip to the physician or laboraory is in order. Following an incubation of 18 to 24 hours, the culture plate reveals the presence or absence of strep.

Treatment

It's foolhardy to treat a troublesome throat infection without a culture. Once the results of the throat culture are known, rational therapy can begin. Streptococcal throat infections require antibiotic therapy for 10 days. Penicillin is the traditional choice of drug, although the physician may prescribe erythromycin (Ilosone) or another antibiotic. Following the 10 days of therapy, a repeat throat culture confirms the success of therapy and the absence of streptococci.

Nonstreptococcal throat infections are caused by a mixed bag of viral and bacterial organisms. Staphylococci and pneumococci may be present, and the physician may prescribe a four- or five-day course of penicillin or mycin drugs to eradicate these organisms, even in the absence of a strep infection.

Many nonprescription medications are available to relieve throat soreness, and these may be the only treatment needed for nonstreptococcal throat infections. Least expensive and highly effective is a warm salt-water gargle four times daily: Dissolve one-half teaspoonful of ordinary table salt in eight ounces of warm-to-hot tap water. Six or eight good gargles will empty the glass, and this procedure is repeated four times daily.

Throat lozenges relieve discomfort and soothe irritated membranes. Here are three good choices:

- Chloraseptic Lozenges, containing menthol, phenol and thymol.
- Phe-Mer-Nite Throat Tablets, containing benzocaine as a local anesthetic, and the germicide phenylmercuric nitrate.
- Thantis Lozenges, containing the anesthetic saligenin and merodicein as an antiseptic.

Although all antibiotics require prescriptions, virtually all throat lozenges or troches are sold over-the-counter, and if the physician prescribes a topical throat medication, you'll save money if it is purchased without prescription.

THROMBOANGIITIS OBLITERANS

Synonym: Buerger's disease

Usually striking a middle-aged Jewish chain-smoker, Buerger's disease causes blood clots in the arteries (in contrast to venous blood clots of phlebitis). The clot blocks blood flow in the artery, and the impaired blood supply causes tissue damage, often progressing to gangrene, that is most noticeable in the extremities.

If untreated, the disease progresses, and amputation of gangrenous limbs may be needed.

The most important aspect of therapy is cessation of smoking. In most cases, stopping smoking stops progression of the disease, while continuing tobacco use leads to progressive blood clots with tissue loss.

Stopping smoking is often all the therapy needed, although the physician may prescribe medication to improve arterial blood flow and/or reduce clotting within the arteries.

THROMBOPHLEBITIS

Synonyms: blood clot in the vein, phlebitis of the veins

The veins of the legs return blood to the body after it has nourished the lower legs and feet. Uniquely adapted to their function, the leg veins utilize the muscular motion of activity to propel the blood uphill against gravity. They even have valves to prevent backflow.

Phlebitis occurs when blood flow in the veins is impeded—perhaps by swelling of the upper thigh, a blockage in the pelvis, or by inactivity that slows the return of venous blood. Trauma may be a factor; phlebitis can follow an injury to the lower extremities. Blood clots in the legs are common following surgery or a heart attack—or any condition necessitating bed rest. Medication can be a factor, and oral contraceptives increase the risk of thrombophlebitis in the lower extremities.

Two types of phlebitis occur: inflammation of the superficial veins under the skin and the more treacherous thrombophlebitis of the deep veins.

Superficial Thrombophlebitis

Inflammation and clotting of the superficial leg veins usually occur below the knee. Local pain is present, associated with swelling, tenderness, and warmth. Rest is advised, and when walking the patient should use well-fitted surgical hose. As with any inflammation, phlebitis of the legs often responds to heat; moist heat is the preferred method, applied as hot packs for one hour four times daily.

In addition, the doctor may prescribe a medication to relieve local inflammation, perhaps phenylbutazone (Butazoladin Alka) capsules taken four times daily with meals.

Superficial thrombophlebitis usually responds to treatment within a few weeks, but often recurs particularly following enforced bed rest or prolonged vigorous activity. If phlebitis of the superficial veins occurs with contraceptives, the use of birth control pills should be stopped.

Thrombophlebitis of the Deep Veins

Phlebitis of the deep veins of the legs causes pain and swelling in the calf. Pressure on the gastrocnemius (calf) muscles causes discomfort, as does forceful upper pressure on the foot. A measurable enlargement and warmth of the lower leg is often present.

Thrombophlebitis of the deep veins of the leg is treacherous, and may send a blood clot suddenly speeding to the heart and lungs.

The physician will advise bed rest plus applications of heat. Hospitalization is sometimes required. Often recommended is anticoagulation, "thinning the blood," using warfarin (Coumadin) to retard blood clotting, but requiring regular blood tests to assess the progress of therapy.

As therapy progresses, the patient will be fitted for tight-fitting surgical hose extending from toe to groin, or perhaps pantyhose for women. Most effective (and most expensive) are the Jobst Surgical Hose, made to exact measurements and donned in the morning before standing—before blood fills the veins.

Thrombophlebitis of the deep veins often causes permanent

valve damage, and after recovery from the acute episode, swelling and a heavy feeling in the leg may be noted at the day's end.

THYROID DISORDERS

Synonyms: hyperthyroidism, hypothroidism, goiter

The thyroid gland, located in the neck, sets the pace for the other organs of the body. Weighing barely an ounce or two, the thyroid gland plays a vital role in metabolism at all levels. When too much thyroid hormone is produced, overactivity of body organs occurs; but a deficient production of thyroid hormone results in sluggishness.

Hypothyroidism

Impaired thyroid production may be associated with an enlarged thyroid (called a goiter and shown in Figure 32). When the body's cells lack thyroid hormones, the gland often enlarges in a valiant effort to produce more circulating thyroid hormone. Symptoms include mental sluggishness, weight gain, dry coarse hair, and puffiness of the face. Constipation is common, and women sufferers may complain of menstrual irregularity.

A thyroid deficiency may result from a poor intake of iodine—a vital component of thyroid hormone. But in these modern times when iodized table salt is in common use, a thyroid deficiency more often results from the gland's inability to meet the body's needs. One common cause is thyroidectomy, with a thyroid deficiency developing years or decades following thyroid surgery to correct a previously overactive throid.

Sometimes newborn infants suffer a congenital thyroid deficiency, resulting in lassitude, facial puffiness, and poor mental function (called cretinism), but the more common picture is the adult with sluggishness and weight gain. When advanced, the disease is called myxedema.

Hypothyroidism can sometimes be prevented by the use of iodized table salt, and this is the only worthwhile self-help measure. When clinical hypothyroidism is present, medical consultation is mandatory. After appropriate testing, the

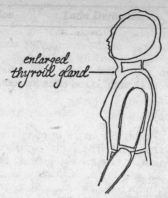

FIGURE 32. *Enlarged thyroid gland.*

physician will prescribe thyroid hormone replacement, perhaps as thyroid extract or in a synthetic compound such as liothyronine (Cytomel), levothyroxine (Synthroid), or liothrix (Euthroid).

Once a thyroid deficiency has been demonstrated, most patients must take supplementary thyroid hormone for life.

Hyperthyroidism

Hyperthyroidism, which may or may not cause enlargement of the gland, produces characteristic symptoms including anxiety, a fine tremor of the hands, weight loss despite a voracious appetite, and perhaps bulging of the eyes. The doctor will note warm fingertips, a bounding blood pressure, rapid pulse, and brisk reflexes. In advanced cases, heart failure or fibrillation (a rapid irregular heartbeat) may occur.

Three possible treatments are available for hyperthyroidism:

- Surgery is the time-honored treatment, with removal of part of the thyroid gland. The surgeon leaves what he estimates to be just enough gland for optimum hormone production.
- Radioiodine administration destroys part of the thyroid gland, and the dose given is carefully calculated to preserve enough thyroid tissue for efficient func-

tion. This method is often recommended for patients who are poor surgical risks, and is most commonly employed in persons over age 40.

- Antithyroid drugs such as propylthiouracil directly combat thyroid overactivity and are often prescribed for children and young adults. The usual course of therapy is 6 to 18 months and often longer.

Thyroid Tumors

A lump in the thyroid, like lumps in other areas, must be considered a cancer suspect. The doctor will order a radio-iodine uptake and scan, to determine if the mass produces thyroid hormone (a hot nodule) or is inactive (a cold nodule, more likely to be cancer). Suspicious nodules are surgically removed and 10 to 12 percent will be found to harbor cancer.

TONSILLITIS

Synonym: tonsil infection

Tonsillitis is a throat infection that strikes the tonsils—those knots of lymphoid tissue that flank the throat. Pockets of pus are often seen, high fever is usually present, and vomiting is not uncommon. In general, tonsillitis is a disease of children, since tonsils shrink in size following puberty. Except for these facts, tonsillitis causes similar symptoms, requires a throat culture, and should be treated the same as other throat infections *(q.v.)*. Strep infections occur in one-quarter or more of all infected tonsils, and demand 10 days of antibiotic treatment once culture confirms the diagnosis.

How About Tonsillectomy?

Removal of the tonsils is sometimes advised. The tonsils are surgically excised, and adenoids are often removed at the same time. Certainly tonsils play a role in preventing disease, and these organs should be sacrificed only when they become a liability, when the discomfort and dangers of recurrent tonsil infections outweigh the potential benefits of retaining the tonsils.

The doctor may recommend tonsillectomy when a youngster suffers four or more throat or ear infections within one year. The case for tonsillectomy is strengthened when the youngster snores at night, suffers habitual mouth breathing during the day, exhibits difficulty swallowing food morsels because of huge tonsils, and show a failure to gain weight and thrive. When advised, tonsillectomy is best performed after the fourth birthday, although the operation may be undertaken earlier when tonsillitis recurs again and again.

One word of caution: Tonsillectomy will not prevent common colds, and removal of the tonsils for no better reason than recurrent colds will only leave a tonsil-less child who still suffers frequent common colds.

TRICHINOSIS

Synonym: measly pork

The Trichinella spiralis is a parasite sometimes found in undercooked pork products, including ham, sausage, pork roast, and so forth. If infected pork is eaten, disease may follow, causing nausea, vomiting, diarrhea, fever, swelling of the face, and a high level of eosinophiles (a type of white blood cell) in the blood. Muscle biopsy clinches the diagnosis when Trichinellae are found in the patient's muscle tissue.

What to Do about Trichinosis

Trichinosis therapy leaves much to be desired. Cortisone may be prescribed, as well as symptomatic treatment, including aspirin and fluids.

Prevention is the keynote. Only government-inspected swine products should be purchased, and buying uninspected pork from a local farmer may mean risking trichinosis. All pork products should be thoroughly cooked. Restaurant sausage that is pink inside should be returned, while pork roasts and ham must be cooked long enough so that all possible infectious organisms are eradicated.

TUBERCULOSIS

Synonyms: consumption, phthisis, TB

We are winning the battle against tuberculosis, but the war is not over yet. Each month, here and there across the United States, a few more cases of tuberculosis are found. Sometimes it's an oldster with a chronic cough, occasionally a child with enlarged lymph glands in the neck. We were not always so lucky.

A half-century ago, tuberculosis was a leading cause of death in this country, and therapy consisted merely of vitamins, a nutritious diet, fresh air, and isolation from healthy individuals. Mortality from tuberculosis fell abruptly following the introduction of anti-TB drugs in 1945. Over the past few decades, widespread use of chest x-rays and tuberculin testing have made great strides against the disease, detecting many cases during early stages when therapy is easier than in the advanced disease.

Tuberculosis is an infectious disease caused by the tubercle bacilli, transmitted by droplets (notably from coughing), as well as via linen, utensils, food, or milk. Although some cases affect the intestine, and infected youngsters often show enlarged neck glands, most initial tuberculosis disease occurs in the lung. When this happens, the body rushes to subdue the TB germs, and most initial infections leave merely a small scar seen on x-ray.

Sometimes the first infection is overwhelming, and in other cases, a later dose of TB germs may overcome defenses. Then severe coughing results, perhaps associated with fever and the formation of a lung cavity. In some individuals tuberculosis spreads to the bones, joints, kidneys, or lymph glands.

Detecting Tuberculosis

Early detection and prompt treatment is the goal of current anti-TB programs. Routine chest x-rays can spot infection even before symptoms begin and can pinpoint those individuals who need further testing.

Tuberculin skin tests (including the widely used tine test) detect past or present TB infection. Read two to three days following its application, a positive TB test means that past or present TB germs have evoked antibodies against the disease; it does not tell if the infection is presently active. A negative tuberculin test is also informative, showing that you have not now nor ever had a TB infection. (One exception to this generality might be the uncommon occurrence of a negative skin test in the victim of an overwhelming TB infection.)

The diagnosis of tuberculosis is confirmed by finding the TB germs on smear and culture. Coughing patients often raise tubercule bacilli in the sputum, but sometimes (particularly in youngsters) the bacteria are obtained by pumping the stomach to obtain swallowed sputum.

Preventing Tuberculosis

Those in contact with a known tuberculosis patient are unlikely to contract the disease from him or her; you catch TB from those who don't know they have it. Of course, the clothing, linen, dishes, utensils, and tissues of active TB patients should be segregated and sterilized. Tissue and other paper goods that may bear infection should be burned. If the patient is coughing, attendants should wear protective masks. Yet, with proper care and frequent hand washing, the risk of infection from a known TB source is minimal.

A vaccine is available. It's called the BCG vaccination, named for the doctors who first developed this weakened strain of tubercle bacilli: Doctors Calmette and Guerin. BCG vaccination acts as a mild infection, building antibodies against tuberculosis. But there is a major drawback: BCG vaccination produces a positive skin test against tuberculosis that persists for perhaps a decade, eliminating the usefulness of this diagnostic procedure during that time.

Drug Treatment of TB

Drug therapy is now the mainstay of tuberculosis treatment, and prolonged sanitarium confinement has become a thing of the past. If tuberculosis is diagnosed, or even strongly suspected, the doctor may recommend treatment with one or more of the following drugs:

- Isoniazid is the most widely used anti-TB drug. It is prescribed when a positive TB skin test is discovered in an infant or in an individual whose tuberculin skin test has converted from negative to positive within the last six months. The doctor may also prescribe pyridoxine (Vitamin B_6) to prevent side effects.

- Rifampin is a recent addition to the anti-TB arsenal. Low white blood counts and liver disease are worrisome side effects.
- Streptomycin is an old-line anti-TB drug. Nerve damage to the ear is a danger and Streptomycin may cause dizziness or ringing in the ears.
- Para-amino Salicylic Acid (PAS), taken in large doses, augments the actions of isoniazid.
- Ethambutol is sometimes substituted for PAS.
- Cycloserine, prescribed less often than several other anti-TB drugs, can cause mental disturbances and convulsions.
- Ethionamide, also not often prescribed, has a relatively high incidence of side effects.

For further information about tuberculosis detection and therapy write to:

National Tuberculosis and Respiratory Disease Association
1740 Broadway
New York, New York 10019

UPPER RESPIRATORY INFECTION

Synonyms: common cold, cold virus

The common cold is aptly named; it's the most frequently occurring afflication of civilized man, striking adults two or three times yearly and children even more often. Even the symptoms are common: there's nothing elegant about nasal congestion, fever, a scratchy throat, and hacking cough. Yes, the cold is indeed a common illness; yet it is one that's uncommonly hard to cure, resisting the most powerful antibiotics and usually lingering for a week or more before subsiding.

Self-help treatment should be the chief attack against the common cold. There's little point in wasting the doctor's time and your money in an office call when most medicines that the doctor may prescribe can be purchased without prescription under different brand names.

When treating the common cold, begin with basics: first, rest at home for a few days if possible. This means sleeping in during the morning, perhaps a nap in the afternoon, and to bed early at night. Take lots of fluids, including fruit juice for vitamins, plus soup and tea to help dissolve thick sticky phlegm. A natural remedy for cold and cough is tea made from horehound leaves. The aches and pains of a common cold respond to aspirin or Bufferin, two tablets every six to eight hours if needed.

Once you have undertaken these fundamental measures, it's time to think about drug treatment. There's a vast array of cold remedies available without prescription. The watchword is: Choose wisely; understand what each medicine is intended to do, and choose the product likely to relieve your symptoms.

Over-The-Counter Cold Remedies

Whatever the sumptoms of your cold, there is a medicine for you in the pharmacy. Analyze your particular cold complaints, and choose products sensibly. The lists below are far from comprehensive, but rather give good choices from the many therapeutic possibilities available.

Congestion characterizes the common cold, with stuffiness, sinus pressure, and an annoying postnasal drip. The treatment of choice is an antihistamine-decongestant combination such as:

- Coricidin D Tablets containing phenylephrine as a decongestant, the antihistamine chlorpheniramine, aspirin, and caffeine.
- Contac Capsules with phenylpropanolamine hydrochloride as the decongestant, chlorpheniramine as an antihistamine, and belladonna alkaloids as drying agents, all packed in a handy time-disintegration capsule.
- Ornex Decongestant Capsules, ideal for individuals who become drowsy with antihistamines. Each capsule contains the decongestant pheylpropanolamine plus the analgesic acetaminophen.

315

Nasal stuffiness can be a most annoying symptom, compromising normal breathing and interfering with sleep. Useful preparations to clear congested noses include:

- Dristan Decongestant Nasal Mist, containing pheniramine maleate, phenylephrine, and benzalkonium chloride.
- Nasocon Nasal Spray containing naphazoline and antazoline.
- Privine Nasal Spray and Drops containing naphazoline.

Perhaps the problem is cough, with a tickling throat irritation, a hacking bark, or a deep, provocative whoop that banishes sleep. Whatever the cough, one of the following preparations is likely to help:

- Cheracol-D Cough Syrup contains glyceryl guaiacolate, dextromethorphan, ammonium chloride, antimony and potassium tartrates, chloroform, and alcohol.
- Consotuss Syrup, long one of my favorites, contains doxylamine, glyceryl guaiacolate, dextromethorphan, chloroform, and alcohol.
- Vicks Formula 44 Extra-Strength Cough Mixture contains doxylamine, sodium citrate, dextromethorphan, chloroform, and 10 percent alcohol.
- NyQuil Liquid, a first-rate choice for nighttime cough, contains doxylamine, dextromethorphan, ephedrine, acetaminophen, and a full 25 percent alcohol.

An irritated throat can be uncomfortable, and may cause recurrent coughing. When this happens, self-help can save the day:

- Anise mint is an old-fashioned remedy for sore throat.
- Chloraseptic Lozenges contain phenol, menthol, and thymol.
- Thantis Lozenges contain saligenin as a topical anesthetic, and the antiseptic merodicein.
- Spec-T Antibacterial Troches contain cetylpyridinium with the local anesthetic benzocaine to calm a tickling throat.

316

Vitamin C and the Common Cold

Large doses of natural Vitamin C help prevent colds. Good sources are oranges and parsley. In fact, when orange juice was unavailable during World War II, British children were given parsley tea to maintain their level of Vitamins A and C.

The last line in the story of Vitamin C and the common cold has yet to be written. Nobel Prize-winning scientist Linus Pauling began a controversy with his book *Vitamin C and the Common Cold* (W. H. Freeman and Company, 1970, reprinted by Bantam Books).

Doctors across America said, "Not true." But here and there a word was heard in defense of Vitamin C.

For example, a study from Ireland shows a change in Vitamin C metabolism during colds, and a Toronto, Canada, scientist told of 1,000 volunteers who received Vitamin C or placebo; although both groups had the same number of colds, the treated group seemed to suffer less and missed fewer days from work.

In his book, Linus Pauling recommended prophylactic doses of Vitamin C to help ward off winter colds. Citing "biochemical individuality," he first pegged his average dose at 1,000 mg to 2,000 mg per day, with a possible range between 250 mg and 5,000 mg. However, in a March 1974 article in *Medical Counterpoint*, Dr. Pauling recommended a lower prophylactic dose of 200 to 1,000 mg.

Does it help? I really don't know, but in time we family doctors may have to admit that Linus Pauling was right, if scientific evidence accumulates to confirm the Vitamin C-common cold treatment.

Treating Children's Colds

One of the great medical pioneers, Bela Schick, once said, "Children are not simply micro-adults, but have their own specific problems." So it is with children's colds. Kids have higher fevers, runnier noses, and appear infinitely sicker than the adult with a comparable cold.

While youngsters with raging fevers, severe coughs, and other signs of severe illness should be examined by the physician, the child with simple nasal congestion, slight cough, a no real fever may respond to the following remedies:

- Novahistine Elixir containing phenylephrine decongestant, the antihistamine chlorpheniramine, and chloroform for cough, all in a 5-percent alcohol base.
- Children's Romilar Cough Syrup containing glyceryl guaiacolate, citric acid, and sodium citrate as expectorants, and dextromethorphan to suppress unnecessary cough.
- One-quarter percent Neo-Synephrine Nasal Spray containing phenylephrine hydrochloride solution.
- Vick's VapoRub, a favorite of several generations of mothers, containing menthol, camphor, spirits of turpentine, cedar leaf oil, nutmeg oil, eucalyptus oil, and thymol—imparting a soothing warmth to the chest as vapors open clogged nasal passages.

Mother's presence lends reassurance, too.

URINARY TRACT INFECTION

Synonyms: cystitis, pyelitis, bladder infection, kidney infection

Urinary tract infections—especially bladder infections—occur most commonly in women since the female anatomy allows relatively easy migration of bacteria from the vagina into the bladder. Once bacteria reach the safe haven of the bladder, they multiply like rabbits, and soon produce cystitis symptoms of bladder irritation and a burning sensation during urination, day and night. Sometimes there is blood in the urine due to a severe irritation of the bladder wall, and infection may arise in one or both kidneys, causing back pain and bounding fever. Common at all ages, cystitis of the female bladder reaches a peak during the sexually active years, when the local trauma of coitus forces bacteria from the vagina up into the bladder. The male anatomy prevents such easy entry, and cystitis in the male is a much less common occurrence than in the female.

Treatment

Cystitis calls for antibacterial therapy, and that means a trip to the doctor. He will probably prescribe a sulfonamide such as Gantrisin, or perhaps tetracycline (Achromycin), ampicillin (Polycillin), nitrofurantoin (Furadantin), nalidixic acid, (NegGram), or trimethoprim-sulfamethoxazole combination (Bactrim or Septra).

If urinary burning is overwhelming, ask the physician for a separate prescription for phenazopyridine (Pyridium), which has the twin properties of alleviating urinary irritation and turning the urine a brilliant orange hue.

Self-help cystitis remedies aim to relieve symptoms and prevent recurrences:

- Drinking lots of water maintains dilute urine and may relieve irritating burning; alcohol and probably coffee should be avoided since they may cause bladder irritation.
- Change the diapers of infants as soon as they are moist.
- Infants with an unexplained fever should be suspected of a bladder infection. Make note of how often urine is passed, since bladder infections cause the frequent elimination of small amounts of urine.
- If bed-wetting (q.v.) persists past age five, the youngster should be checked by a urologist; a structural abnormality may be the cause of recurrent infections in the urinary tract.
- Women who note that bladder infections often coincide with vaginal irritation should seek definitive treatment of the vaginal disorder, and I advise these women to cease the use of tampons for six months. Tampons in the vagina stimulate inflammation as the body tries to eliminate the foreign object. Use pads instead, and less vaginal irritation may mean fewer bladder infections.
- If severe bladder irritation seems to prevent the passage of urine, sit in a tub of hot water. If this fails to promote urinary passage, relief may follow an effort to pass the urine directly into the bath water. It

sounds unpleasant, but it's better than having tubes inserted into your urinary tract.

- Recurrent bladder infections and irritation are sometimes alleviated by taking two six-ounce glasses of cranberry juice each day.
- Women who suffer frequent cystitis following sexual relations sometimes can prevent infection by taking a one-day course of sulfa or other antibiotic following coitus. Also helpful is passing urine immediately after the sexual encounter, washing bacteria out of the bladder.
- Finally, bladder infections are too serious to be trusted to over-the-counter preparations. Urinary antiseptics, "kidney pills," and the rest just won't do the job when bladder infection strikes, and may result in a dangerous delay of effective treatment. When bladder symptoms of burning and frequent urination are present, call the doctor—and fast.

VAGINITIS

Synonyms: vaginal infection, including trichomoniasis, candidiasis, moniliasis, yeast infection, and non-specific vaginitis

Although almost all vaginal infections cause local pain, burning, itching, and discharge, there are several distinct types of infections, treated in different ways.

Some mucus discharge from the vagina is normal and, in fact, the vagina is normally inhabited by "resident" germs of various types. All is in balance until one of these inhabitants begins to multiply and outstrips the others to cause the symptoms of infection. Factors that can upset the vaginal ecology are:

- Lowered resistance to infection due to poor diet or lack of sleep.
- The presence of other disease such as flu.
- A change in vaginal acidity due to pregnancy or oral contraceptives.
- A reaction to intravaginal tampons.
- Irritation due to excessive douching.

320

- Death of "good germs" following antibiotic use.
- Some causes we haven't learned about yet.

The Types of Vaginitis

Three types of vaginitis occur, and accurate diagnosis requires a pelvic examination with microscopic examination and culture of the discharge.

Trichomonal infections, due to Trichomonas vaginalis, cause vaginal irritation and a malodorous thin discharge. On microscopic examination, the doctor can see the small active parasites darting about. Therapy should include metronidazole (Flagyl) tablets and vaginal inserts for both the patient and her mate. During the 10-day course of treatment a condom should be used during sexual relations.

Monilial or Candida vaginitis is due to a yeast fungus called Candida albicans. Severe vaginal discomfort, especially during sex relations, is associated with a thick cheesy discharge. The diagnosis is confirmed by culture and the treatment is miconazole (Monistat) cream or nystatin (Mycostatin) vaginal tablets used twice daily for three weeks. Monilial infections often follow antibiotic use and several young women have reported that a yogurt douche has prophylactic value and can abort early symptoms.

Bacterial infections also cause a vaginal discharge and discomfort. The possibility of gonorrheal infection must be considered, and this is discussed on page 137. However, most bacterial vaginitis is caused by Hemophilus vaginalis, diagnosed on microscopic examination, and treated with sulfonamide (Sultrin) vaginal tablets or cream.

Sometimes several types of infections coexist; the diagnosis is then nonspecific vaginitis and combination treatment is required.

Prevention and Treatment

Although specific medication is the best therapy for vaginal infections, the following self-help program can aid prevention:

- Maintain the best health possible, with a nutritious diet, lots of exercise, and adequate rest.
- Avoid layers of tight-fitting undergarments, especially

321

- synthetic fibers, that can create a warm, moist haven for germs.
- Many germs that cause vaginitis are present in the rectum. After a bowel movement, always wipe front to back, and teach your daughters this technique.
- Be wary of medication, especially antibiotics and estrogens. Many doctors prescribe prophylactic vaginal medication if the vaginitis-prone woman must take penicillin or tetracycline.
- Consider tampons a possible course of irritation. Sometimes recurrent vaginitis is relieved only by a switch from tampons to pads.
- Sexual partners can carry infection without symptoms, and males often require treatment.
- Avoid sexual intercourse when discomfort is at its worst, and a condom should be used in any sexual relations during the course of therapy.
- Minimal vaginal irritation and/or discharge may respond to a vinegar douche, using one ounce of white vinegar per quart of warm water. However, for persistent or severe symptoms see the doctor.
- Always finish any prescribed course of medication and keep any follow-up appointment, even if symptoms are relieved. Many instances of recurrent vaginitis are related to treatment stopped too soon.

There is a good book available. Ask your doctor for the booklet *For Your Information . . . Vaginitis* published by Ortho Pharmaceutical Corporation, Raritan, New Jersey 08869.

VARICOCELE

An enlargement of the scrotal veins is called a varicocele, often encountered in schoolboys and older men. Usually there are no symptoms, and the varicocele looks and feels like a "bag of worms" on the left side of the scrotum (see Figure 33). For anatomical reasons, virtually all varicoceles are left-sided, and a right-sided engorgement of the scrotal veins suggests that a causative disease may be present; see the doctor.

The varicocele causes few symptoms, although an occasional male describes a dull ache in the scrotum. Chronicity is the rule, although some teenage varicoceles disappear later in life.

No therapy is needed for this harmless variant—if no symptoms are present. The boy or man who complains of vague discomfort may find relief wearing snug Jockey shorts or even a scrotal sling.

Reassurance is important, lest the patient confuse a harmless varicocele with more serious scrotal disorders.

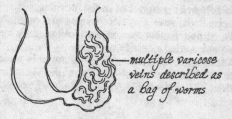

multiple varicose veins described as a bag of worms

FIGURE 33. *Left varicocele.*

VARICOSE VEINS

Synonyms: swollen veins of the legs, venous varicosities

The veins of the legs carry blood from the lower extremities back into the body. Lacking the forceful cardiac thrust of arterial blood flow, the leg veins convey blood "uphill" against gravity by utilizing muscular contraction of the legs plus a series of valves to prevent backflow. Varicose veins—swelling of the venous channels of the legs—begin as blood pools in the vessels. A family history of this defect is common, and predisposing factors include obesity, pregnancy, phlebitis of the legs, tight encircling garters, and anything that impedes blood flow through the leg veins.

What to Do about Varicose Veins

Avoid pooling of blood in the veins through regular exercise (including walking and running) alternating with rest periods with the legs elevated. The muscular contraction of exercise stimulates blood flow in the veins, while elevation of the feet allows the veins to drain by gravity.

Fat persons should lose weight, and the woman with severe varicose veins must consider the hazards imposed by any contemplated pregnancy. Tight encircling garments are avoided, since that can block venous blood flow.

Compression dressings help. Ace Elastic Bandages, four to six inches in width, are often used, although surgical hose eliminate the frequent adjustments needed with elastic bandages. Most efficient are Jobst Elastic Stockings, made to order from multiple measurements of the extremities and applied before arising from bed in the morning.

If all else fails, severe varicose veins are often "stripped" surgically, although new venous varicosities may re-form in remaining veins after a decade or two.

Those interested in learning more about this topic can request the booklet *Varicose Veins* from the American Heart Association, 7320 Greenville Avenue, Dallas, Texas 75231.

VIRAL GASTROENTERITIS

Synonyms: gastroenteritis, viral intestinal flu, diarrhea

Common viral gastroenteritis strikes everyone from time to time, including tiny infants and strong laborers. Abdominal cramps, vomiting, and/or diarrhea may occur, together with loss of appetite, lassitude, and perhaps a low-grade fever. One or more symptoms may predominate, and manifestations may differ in various family members who have contracted the disease. One individual may suffer severe vomiting, while the next complains of profuse diarrhea.

Viral gastroenteritis is a self-limited condition; no matter what you do it goes away, and there is no definite cure. Treatment is directed toward relieving symptoms, not only to make the sufferer more comfortable, but to prevent dehydration.

Treatment

Whether the chief complaint is vomiting or diarrhea, it's best to take plenty of fluids for a few days. Although solids may be eaten if the appetite permits, the gastroenteritis sufferer should take a high-liquid diet including:

Water at room temperature
Thin soup
Weak tea
Ginger ale
Kool-aid and Popsicles for youngsters
Boiled skimmed milk
Dilute fruit juice.

Barley water is a good home remedy for diarrhea: boil five cupfuls of water, to which is added one cupful of grain barley. Simmer the mixture 20 to 30 minutes, then strain off the fluid. Drink three to four cupfuls of this barley water daily until diarrhea subsides.

Vomiting often responds to nonprescription Emetrol, an oral solution containing dextrose, levulose, and orthophosphoric acid. The dose for infants and children is one or two teaspoonfuls at 15-minute intervals until vomiting ceases; adults take one or two tablespoonfuls in the same manner. If the first dose is vomited, wait five minutes, then try again.

Diarrhea is treated with kaolin and pectin, perhaps accompanied by belladonna derivatives to slow intestinal motility. No prescription is needed for:

• Donnagel, containing kaolin, hyoscyamine, atropine, and hyoscine.
• Kao-Con, a concentrated solution of kaolin and pectin.
• Kaopectate, a kaolin-pectin combination favored by patients for generations.

These measures usually suffice, and within a few days improvement is evident. However, if vomiting is relentless and diarrhea unchecked, it's time to call the physician.

VITAMIN DEFICIENCIES

Synonym: avitaminosis
Vitamin deficiencies today are, like high-button shoes and

horse-drawn carriages, of historical significance. Of course, there's an exception here and there—the rare Vitamin D-deficient infant with bony rickets, the snack-food teen-ager with subclinical malnutrition, or the oldster with Vitamin B deficiencies following a tea-and-toast diet. Yet despite the abundance of vitamins in our diet, vitamin supplements enjoy multimillion dollar sales and interest in these simple biochemical entities flourishes.

Vitamins are an odd assortment of chemical compounds participating in vital metabolic reactions within the body. Without this vitamin or that, a basic chemical reaction fails to take place and disease ensues. Over the years, we have been able to determine the chemical function and daily requirements of some well-known vitamins, while others remain shrouded in mystery.

Vitamin A deficiency causes impaired vision in subdued light, called night blindness, associated with irritation of the outer layer of the eye and sometimes with skin disorders. Related to carotene pigment (the yellow color of carrots and similar yellow vegetables), Vitamin A occurs abundantly in fish oils, liver, eggs, milk, butter, and, of course, vegetables. The recommended daily allowance for adults is 5,000 units, easily exceeded by the usual diet since one egg contains 600 international units, a cup of beef stew contains more than 2,-000 international units, and two ounces of fried beef liver bursts with 30,000 international units. In fact, individuals popping vitamins pills by the handful are in danger of developing *hyper*vitaminosis A, observed when 75,000 to 500,-000 international units of Vitamin A are consumed for a prolonged period of time, and causing sores of the skin, headache, neuritis, blurred vision, and vomiting.

Vitamin D controls the metabolism of calcium and its deposition in bone. Ultraviolet rays of the sun spur endogenous (produced within the body) Vitamin D production in the skin, but the best source is cod or halibut liver oil. In America, most milk is fortified with 400 international units of Vitamin D per quart—the recommended daily dietary allowance of this vital nutrient. Vitamin D, like Vitamins A and E, is dissolved by fat and deficiency may follow impaired food absorption due to bile obstruction or overuse of mineral oil laxatives.

Vitamin C (ascorbic acid) has a colorful history. Ancient writings and records of the Crusades describe the weakness, skin sores, and swollen gums of scurvy; and the disease became an occupational hazard of sailors on long voyages. When Vasco da Gama sailed around the Cape of Good Hope in 1498, 100 of his crew of 160 men died of scurvy during the voyage. Then, in 1747, British naval surgeon James Lind studied the effects of citrus fruits on scurvy, prescribing for the afflicted two oranges and one lemon every day. Following his dramatic experiments, the daily ingestion of citrus fruits became mandatory for the British sailor, earning him to this day the nickname Limey. Milk products have only 2 to 5 mg of ascorbic acid per serving, each serving of meat has no more, a vegetable serving will have roughly 20 mg. while eight ounces of orange juice has more than 100 mg of ascorbic acid, well exceeding the recommended adult daily dietary allowance of 60 mg of Vitamin C.

Vitamin B_1 (thiamine) aids the metabolism of carbohydrates and a deficiency leads to a disorder of the nerves classically known as beriberi. Beriberi occurred in epidemics throughout Southeast Asia until scientists proved that birds fed polished rice developed the disease and could be cured by eating the unpolished grain. By removing the kernels from the grain that was the staple of their diets, Orientals were discarding the vitamin-rich portion. When this practice stopped, beriberi disappeared. The recommended adult daily allowance is 1.0 to 1.4 mg, and the best sources are whole grains, yeast, vegetables, and meat.

Vitamin B_2 (riboflavin) aids the metabolism of many foods, and is found in meat, liver, cheese, eggs, and milk products. A Vitamin B_2 deficiency, called ariboflavinosis, occurs in individuals receiving less than the recommended daily allowance of 1.5 mg, and is characterized by sores at the corner of the mouth and skin rashes.

Niacin (nicotinic acid) shortage causes pellagra, a disease common in the southern United States during the early twentieth century. Rural southerners, consuming a diet high in corn products and molasses, often developed pellagra symptoms of skin rash, diarrhea, and mental disturbances. The pioneering work of Dr. Joseph Goldberger of the United States Public Health Service showed that adding lean beef, milk, and yeast to the diet could cure pellagra. Today, the recommended dietary allowance of niacin is 13 to 20 mg. Vitamin enthusiasts are cautioned to heed this recommendation, since huge amounts of nicotinic acid can cause a bright red flushing of the skin.

Vitamin B_6 (pyridoxine) aids metabolism of proteins and fats. A Vitamin B_6 shortage causes neuritis, oily skin, and occasional convulsions in infants. Tuberculosis patients receiving isoniazide therapy sometimes develop a neuritis responsive to pyridoxine, and recent reports indicate that women taking oral contraceptives sometimes develop a lethargy responsive to Vitamin B_6; both these conditions call for doses greater than the recommended daily allowance of 2.0 mg.

Vitamin K, the coagulation vitamin, is made by bacteria within the intestinal tract. Deficiency, characterized by easy bleeding, may result from a digestive disorder such as sprue, celiac disease, or abuse of oily laxatives. The coumarin anticoagulants interfere with Vitamin K activity, and their blood-thinning action is countered by Vitamin K administration.

Vitamin B_{12} (cyanocobalamin) helps bring red blood cells to maturity and maintains proper nerve function. Vitamin B_{12} occurs abundantly in liver, meat, and dairy products, but its absorption depends upon the presence of "intrinsic factor" in the stomach lining cells. When the intrinisic factor is lacking, Vitamin B_{12} speeds through the intestinal tract without being absorbed and pernicious anemia results, with profound anemia and deterioration of nerves. Vitamin B_{12} injections have long been given as a nonspecific tonic for fatigue, and a *British Journal of Nutrition* report of a study suggests that this beneficial effect may have scientific validity. The recommended daily allowance of Vitamin B_{12} is 5 micrograms, although pernicious anemia sufferers will not respond to many times that amount in the diet and are dependent upon injections of 100 to 1,000 micrograms of Vitamin B_{12} at monthly intervals or less.

Vitamin E (alpha tocopherol) is the everything vitamin: it has been recommended as a cure for more than 100 diseases, and advocates continue to find new indications almost daily. Structurally related to alcohol, Vitamin E plays an obscure metabolic role, and the recommended adult daily allowance of 25 to 30 international units is a "seat-of-the-pants" recommendation based upon the content of foods rather than scientific studies on deficiency states. While the studies of Vitamin E continue, its role remains enigmatic, although true believers continue to consume alpha tocopherol in ever-increasing quantities to alleviate obesity, heart disease, sexual inadequacy, plus a host of other real or imagined ills.

Other vitamins play lesser roles in the metabolic drama: Pantothenic acid deficiencies caused the burning-foot syndrome observed in World War II prisoners in the Far East, relieved by a diet high in pantothenic-acid-containing green and yellow vegetables. A deficiency of folic acid can cause anemia not unlike pernicious anemia, responsive to a diet high in vegetables and liver. And it's noteworthy that folic acid can alleviate the anemia of Vitamin B_{12} deficiency, pernicious anemia, without improving the nerve deficit. A biotin deficiency can be induced by feeding huge quantities of egg white, which binds biotin in the intestines; other than this nutritional curiosity, the adequate quantities of biotin in American foods make this substance of little clinical importance. Finally, there's Vitamin B_{15} (pangamic acid), discovered by E. E. Krebbs in 1965, touted as a treatment for hardened arteries and nerve disorders, and controversial Vitamin B_{17}, described as a potent weapon against cancer.

The story of vitamins, deeply rooted in folklore and shrouded in mystery, can be as exciting as a detective tale. Readers who want to know more will enjoy the books *The Vitamin Pioneers* by Herbert Baily (Rodale Books, Emmaus, Pennsylvania) and *Food for Nought: The Decline in Nutrition* by Ross Hume (Harper & Row, New York).

Vitamin Supplements

The AMA and the FDA often have opposing viewpoints, but they agree on one thing: a balanced American diet containing meat, vegetables, fruit, dairy products (including Vitamin D fortified milk), breads, and cereals provides abundant quantities of all vitamins that we have discussed. Supplementary vitamins are recommended for infants (and these often include fluoride to build strong teeth), for individuals with chronic disease whose dietary intake may be impaired, and for older individuals who may suffer dietary restriction or impaired absorption. Sometimes vitamins are helpful when recovering from a prolonged flu or other illness, and individuals with chronic fatigue often report feeling better when taking a one-a-day vitamin (although this benefit may be more psychological than physical).

If supplementary vitamins are needed, here are some good choices:

- Dayalets Vitamins are small, film-covered, and easily swallowed. They contain:

Vitamin A	5,000 international units
Vitamin D	400 international units
Vitamin C	60 mg
Vitamin B_1	1.5 mg
Vitamin B_2	1.7 mg
Niacin	20 mg
Vitamin B_6	2 mg
Vitamin B_{12}	6 micrograms
Vitamin E	30 international units
Folic acid	0.4 mg

- Dayalets Plus Iron contain the above formula plus 18 mg of ferrous sulfate (iron). The dose of Dayalets or Dayalets Plus Iron is one tablet daily.
- Clusivol Vitamins have the advantage of availability as tablets, capsules, chewable tablets, and tasty syrup for children and oldsters. Each teaspoonful of Clusivol Vitamins contains:

Vitamin A	2,500 international units
Vitamin D	400 international units
Vitamin C	20 mg
Vitamin B_1	1 mg
Vitamin B_2	1 mg
Niacin	5 mg
Vitamin B_6	0.6 mg
Pantothenic acid	3 mg
Vitamin B_{12}	2 micrograms
Iron	3 mg
Manganese	0.5 mg
Zinc	0.5 mg
Magnesium	3.0 mg

  The usual dose of Clusivol Syrup is one teaspoonful daily.
- Feminins Tablets are a vitamin-mineral supplement for women taking oral contraceptives, and each smooth-coated tablet contains:

Vitamin A	5,000 international units
Vitamin D	400 international units
Vitamin C	200 mg
Vitamin B_1	1.5 mg
Vitamin B_2	3 mg
Niacin	15 mg
Vitamin B_6	25 mg
Vitamin B_{12}	10 micrograms
Vitamin E	10 international units
Pantothenic acid	10 mg

Folic acid	0.1 mg
Iron	18 mg
Zinc	10 mg

The usual dose of Feminins Vitamins is one tablet daily.

WARTS

Synonym: verruca

Most of us will develop a wart or two at some time during life, and a few individuals suffer successive crops of verrucae, indicating a special susceptibility to warts. Probably caused by a virus with a low level of contagion, warts may be found on the face, hands, feet, or practically any area of the body. Therapy varies with the location and type of wart present.

Common Wart

Called verucca vulgaris, the common wart can occur on virtually any area of the body. The treatment of common warts is rich in folklore. Grandmothers once advised youngsters to apply stump water by the light of the full moon; the treatment often worked, attesting to the occasional success of suggestion therapy. Natural remedies are often advised: one authority recommends repeated applications of dandelion sap to warts. Castor oil is another folk rememdy for warts, applied directly, once or twice daily, over a period of two to six months.

Small warts, particularly if new and not well entrenched, may respond to local applications of Vergo, which contains calcium pantothenate and ascorbic acid. Widespread warts may be treated in the doctor's office using stronger bichloracetic acid, but the quick, sure wart-removal method is electrocautery by the doctor following the local injection of lidocaine (Xylocaine).

Plantar Warts

The plantar wart (verruca plantaris) is a contagious wart caused by a virus, and often is contracted by teen-agers in swimming pools and shower rooms. Occurring on the sole of the foot, the plantar wart is driven deep into the tissues and extraction is difficult (and painful). Most experts advise against the use of electrocautery on the sole of the foot where a painful scar may result; home therapy is rarely successful; and favored treatment methods include surgical curettage, often used in conjunction with applications of bichloracetic acid by the doctor. Because of the contagious nature of the wart, the patient should avoid walking barefoot in the family bathroom and public areas until pronounced cured.

Flat Warts

The flat wart is called verucca plana, and usually strikes children. Usually multiple and often hard to see, the flat wart may occur on any surface but is usually found on the face or hands. Topical medication as self-help therapy often works, and the preferred agent is Vergo applied in a thin film once daily.

Venereal Wart

The venereal wart is called condyloma acuminatum by the physician, and may affect the male or female genital organs. The growth is contagious and hard to treat, and therapy should be undertaken only by the physician. Often applied is podophyllin in tincture of benzoin or alcohol, a highly caustic compound that can burn the tissues if improperly applied.

WHOOPING COUGH

Synonym: pertussis

Before the widespread use of the whooping cough vaccine a generation ago, pertussis was a common illness of infants and children. Today, thanks to the P (pertussis) of the DPT vaccine (see Immunizations), the disease is as rare as a winter robin, although a sporadic case or even a small epidemic is encountered when the level of community protection falls. In fact, since most children receive pertussis immunizations, this "childhood disease" is now just as likely to be seen in adults.

Caused by a bacteria called Hemophilus pertussis, spread

from person to person by droplets from the respiratory tract, pertussis shows its first symptoms following a two-week incubation period. Once witnessed, pertussis is not forgotten. Initial coughing episodes soon give way to the characteristic whoop—an all-consuming paroxysm of coughing with a red face, protruding tongue, impaired breathing, and the loud high-pitched sound which gives the whoop its name.

What to do about Whooping Cough

Immunization is our best protection. Youngsters should receive DPT injections at two, three, and four months of age with booster injections at two and five years. Because of side effects, it is recommended that pertussis vaccine not be given to individuals age eight and over unless the doctor concludes that the risk of a reaction is outweighed by the possible benefits.

Be suspicious of pertussis. If a common cold causes a cough of increasing severity, coupled with difficulty breathing, see the doctor. And don't be afraid to ask if he thinks it might be whooping cough. If so, he will prescribe intensive antibiotic therapy, along with expectorants and perhaps inhalation therapy. Don't delay long if you suspect whooping cough, since early treatment can speed recovery.

If you want more information about whooping cough or other contagious diseases, write to:

Center for Disease Control
Atlanta, Georgia 30333

Self-Help Appendix

WEIGHT-WATCHER'S CALORIE GUIDE

Food	Approximate Calories
Almonds, 1 dozen	90
Apple, 1 large	100
Applesauce, sweetened, ½ cup	100
Apricots, 10 dried	100
Asparagus, 5 stalks	25
Avocado, 1 average	185
Bacon, 3 slices cooked	100
Banana, 1 medium	90
Beans, canned, ½ cup	175
Beans, lima, ½ cup	100
Beans, snap, ½ cup	25
Beef, lean, 2 ounces	125
Beets, 1 serving (2 small beets)	50
Biscuit, 1 average	100
Blackberries, 1 cup	100
Blueberries, 1 cup	90
Bologna, 1 slice	90
Bread, rye, 1 slice	70
Bread, white, enriched, 1 slice	70
Bread, whole wheat, 1 slice	75
Broccoli, 3 stalks	100
Brownies, 1 average	140
Butter, 1 tablespoon	90
Cabbage, cooked, 1 cup	75
Cake, chocolate or vanilla, no icing	200
with icing, medium slice	250
Cantaloupe, small melon	100
Carrot, 8 inches long	50

```
Cauliflower, ½ cup ............................  25
Celery, 1 stalk ...............................   8
Cheese, cottage, 4 tablespoons .................  80
         cream, 1 tablespoon ..................  55
Cherries, sweet, 10 large ......................  50
Chicken, broiled, ¼ medium broiler ............ 140
         fried, small leg ..................... 65
         roasted, 2 slices .................... 150
Chow Mein, 3½ ounces .......................... 100
Clams, Cherrystone, 6 large ...................  95
Cocoa, all milk (1 cup, 6 ounces milk) ......... 175
         half milk (1 cup, 3 ounces milk) ...... 110
Cola soft drink, 6 ounce bottle ................  75
Corn, ½ cup ...................................  70
Corn flakes, 1 cup ............................  80
Crackers, cheese (1 medium or 10 tiny) .........  20
         Ritz .........................(1)......  15
         Saltine ......................(1)......  15
Cranberry sauce, canned, ½ cup ................ 200
Cream, light, 2 tablespoons ...................  65
         heavy, 2 tablespoons ................. 120
         sour, 1 cup ........................... 455
         whipped, sugar added (1 tablespoon) ...  55
Cucumber, ½ medium ...........................  10

Dates, 10 medium, pitted ...................... 275
Doughnuts, cake, plain, 1 average size ......... 125
         jelly, 1 ............................. 225
         sugared or iced, 1 ................... 150
Duck, roasted, 1 slice ........................ 110

Eggs, 1 medium, boiled ........................  80
      1 medium, fried ......................... 110
      1 medium, scrambled ..................... 100
Eggplant, raw, 2 slices .......................  25
Endive, 20 long leaves ........................  20
Escarole, 10 small leaves .....................   7

Figs, dried, 2 small ..........................  60
Flour, white or whole grain, 1 tablespoon ......  35
Frankfurter, (1) .............................. 125

Gelatin, fruit flavored, prepared, ½ cup .......  85
Ginger ale, 1 cup .............................  80
Grapefruit, ½ medium ..........................  50
Grapes, seedless, 30 ..........................  75
Griddle cakes, 1 medium .......................  75
```

```
Halibut, 1 medium piece .......................  200
Ham, lean, 1 slice ............................  300
Herbs .........................................    0
Honey, 1 tablespoon ...........................   85

Ice Cream, ½ cup ..............................  200
Ice Cream soda, 8 ounces ......................  260
Ice milk, ¼ pint ..............................  100

Jams and jellies, 1 tablespoon ................   60
Juices, orange, fresh, 1 cup ..................  110
        tomato, canned, 1 cup .................   50

Kale, ½ cup, cooked ...........................   50

Lamb, roast, 1 medium slice ...................  100
Lard, 1 tablespoon ............................  100
Lettuce, 2 large leaves .......................    5
Liver, 1 medium slice .........................  100
Liverwurst, 2 ounces ..........................  130
Lobster meat, ½ cup ...........................   75

Macaroni, 1 cup, cooked .......................  150
Macaroni and cheese, 3½ ounces ................  225
Maple syrup, 1 tablespoon .....................   70
Margarine, 1 tablespoon .......................  100
Marshmallow, 1 ................................   20
Mayonnaise, 1 tablespoon ......................  100
Milk, evaporated, 1 cup .......................  180
      instant non-fat dry, 6 tablespoons ......   80
      skim milk, fresh, 1 cup .................   85
      whole milk, 1 cup .......................  160
Mushrooms, 10 large ...........................   10
Mustard, prepared, 1 tablespoon ...............   10

Noodles, ½ cup, cooked ........................   50
Nuts, mixed, 10 ...............................   80

Oatmeal, ½ cup, cooked ........................   75
Oil, corn, cottonseed, olive, peanut, safflower, 1 tbs. ..  100
Onions, 1 medium ..............................   40
Orange, 1 medium ..............................   75

Peaches, canned in syrup, 2 large halves ......  100
         fresh, 1 medium ......................   40
Peanut butter, 1 tablespoon ...................  100
Pears, canned in syrup, 3 halves ..............  100
       fresh, 1 medium ........................   50
```

Peas, canned, ½ cup 65
Pepper, green, 1 medium 20
Pickles, dill, 1 large 10
Pie, 1/6 of pie, apple 410
     custard 325
     lemon meringue 355
     mincemeat 435
     pecan 670
     pumpkin 315
Pineapple, canned, unsweetened, 1 slice 50
Pizza pie, frozen, baked, average piece 250
Plums, 1 fresh 30
Popcorn, plain, 1 cup 55
Pork, 1 lean chop 200
Potato chips, 10 large 110
Potato salad with mayonnaise, ¼ cup 100
Potatoes, baked, 1 large 140
    boiled, 1 medium 75
    french fried, 10 150
    sweet, candied, 1 small 125
Prune juice, ½ cup 100
Prunes, dried, 10 large 250
Radishes, 5 small 10
Raisins, ¼ cup 100
Rice, 1 cup, cooked 125

Salad dressing, 1 tablespoon, French 90
        Italian 75
        Russian 55
Sherbet, ½ cup 120
Spaghetti, 1 cup, cooked 165
Spinach, 1 cup cooked 40
Strawberries, fresh, 1 cup 60
Sugar, brown, granulated, powdered, 1 tablespoon .. 45

Tomatoes, canned, ½ cup or 1 fresh 30
Tuna fish, canned in oil, drained, 1 cup 220
    canned, water pack, 1 cup 130
Turkey, roasted, 2 medium slices 175
Turnip, 1 25

Veal, roast, 1 slice medium size 120

Waffles, 1 medium 200
Walnuts, 10 120
Watermelon, 1 medium slice 200

READING A PRESCRIPTION

The prescription is a legal document ordering a specific medication for a particular patient. Although more than 97 percent of all prescriptions written today are for prepared tablets, capsules, or liquids, the written prescription follows the traditional format evolved generations ago when pharmacists compounded each prescription "from scratch."

A properly written prescription contains eight important parts:

1. The patient's name and address must be noted, including the patient's age if the medication is intended for a child.
2. The date that the prescription was written must always be present, allowing the pharmacist to detect outdated orders.
3. The superscription consists of the symbol Rx (probably derived from the astronomical symbol for Jupiter, the supreme deity of Roman mythology). The Rx symbol is translated as "take thou" and identifies the document as a medical prescription.
4. The inscription describes the medication ordered, including the name and amount of each drug. Whenever possible, generic names and English words should be used in preference to brand names and Latin abbreviations.
5. The subscription is the doctor's instruction to the pharmacist. The subscription may direct the pharmacist to dispense 30 capsules or to combine ingredients into solution.
6. The signature is the doctor's instruction to the patient. Often preceded by the abbreviation Sig. or by the English word Label, the signature directions will be typed by the pharmacist onto the container label. The signature may direct the patient to "Take one

capsule three times daily" or "Apply two drops to each eye every four hours."

7. The refill information is completed for each prescription. In some cases, no refill is allowed. Under federal regulations, depressant and stimulant drugs cannot be refilled more than five times, and the prescription becomes invalid after six months. In some cases, the physician will allow as many as 12 or 20 refills of his prescription.

8. The prescriber's signature completes the prescription and makes it a legal document. If not preprinted on the prescription blank, the physician will add his office address and telephone number.

Here is what a completed prescription form typically looks like:

Henry Smith, M.D.
100 Pine Street
Smalltown, Pa., 12345 .

Telephone—(123) 456-7890

Name: Mary Johnson   Age: 14
Address: 200 Lincoln Street   Date: March 16, 1976
        Smalltown, Pa.

Rx
Buffered penicillin G tablets 400,000 units.
Dispense 20 tablets.

Sig: Take one tablet 4 times daily for 5 days.

Refill 1 time

                                   Henry Smith, M.D.

LATIN PRESCRIPTION PHRASES AND ABBREVIATIONS

Abbreviation	Latin Derivation	English Meaning
aa	ana	of each
a.c.	ante cibum	before meals
ad	ad	to, up to
ad lib.	ad libitum	as desired
aur.	auris	ear
b.i.d.	bis in die	twice a day
bis	bis	twice
c̄	cum	with
caps.	capsula	capsule
d.	dexter	right
d.	dies	day
disp.	dispensa	dispense
f., ft.	fac, fiat	make
gm., Gm., g.	gramma	gram
gr.	grana	grain
gtt.	gutta	drop
h.	hora	hour
h.s.	hora somni	at bedtime
m.	misce	mix
mixt.	mixtura	mixture
no.	numerous	number
non rep.	non repetatur	do not repeat
o.d.	oculus dexter	right eye
o.h.	omni hora	every hour
o.s.	oculus sinister	left eye
o.u.	oculus uterque	each eye
p.c.	post cibum	after meals
p.r.n.	pro re nata	as needed
pulv.	pulvis	powder
q.	quaque	each, every
q.h.	quaque hora	every hour
q.i.d.	quater in die	four times a day
s̄	sine	without
sig.	signa	label
sol.	solutio	solution
s.s.	semi	one-half
stat.	statim	at once
syr.	syrupus	syrup
tab.	tabella	tablet

Abbreviation	Latin Derivation	English Meaning
t.i.d.	ter in die	three times a day
tinct., tr.	tinctura	tincture
ung.	unguentum	ointment
ut dict.	ut dictum	as directed

CONVERSION TABLE: APOTHECARY WEIGHTS AND METRIC EQUIVALENTS

1/600	grain —	0.10 mg		¾	grain —	50 mg
1/500	grain —	0.12 mg		1	grain —	60 mg
1/400	grain —	0.15 mg		1¼	grains —	75 mg
1/300	grain —	0.20 mg		1½	grains —	100 mg
1/250	grain —	0.25 mg		2	grains —	0.12 gm
1/200	grain —	0.30 mg		2½	grains —	0.15 gm
1/150	grain —	0.40 mg		3	grains —	0.20 gm
1/120	grain —	0.50 mg		4	grains —	0.25 gm
1/100	grain —	0.60 mg		5	grains —	0.30 gm
1/80	grain —	0.80 mg		6	grains —	0.40 gm
1/60	grain —	1.0 mg		7½	grains —	0.50 gm
1/50	grain —	1.2 mg		10	grains —	0.60 gm
1/40	grain —	1.5 mg		12	grains —	0.75 gm
1/30	grain —	2.0 mg		15	grains —	1.0 gm
1/20	grain —	3.0 mg		22	grains —	1.5 gm
1/15	grain —	4.0 mg		30	grains —	2.0 gm
1/12	grain —	5.0 mg			(½ dram)	
1/10	grain —	6.0 mg		45	grains —	3.0 gm
1/8	grain —	8.0 mg		60	grains —	4.0 gm
1/6	grain —	10 mg			(1 dram)	
1/5	grain —	12 mg		75	grains —	5.0 gm
¼	grain —	15 mg		90	grains —	6.0 gm
⅓	grain —	20 mg		2	drams —	8.0 gm
⅜	grain —	25 mg		2½	drams —	10 gm
½	grain —	30 mg		4	drams —	15 gm
⅔	grain —	40 mg		1	ounce —	30 gm

CONVERSION TABLE: LIQUID APOTHECARY MEASUREMENTS AND METRIC EQUIVALENTS

½ minim	—	0.03 ml
¾ minim	—	0.05 ml
1 minim	—	0.06 ml
1½ minims	—	0.10 ml
3 minims	—	0.20 ml
4 minims	—	0.25 ml
5 minims	—	0.30 ml
8 minims	—	0.50 ml
10 minims	—	0.60 ml
12 minims	—	0.75 ml
15 minims	—	1.0 ml
30 minims	—	2.0 ml
45 minims	—	3.0 ml
1 fluid dram	—	4 ml
1¼ fluid drams	—	5 ml
2 fluid drams	—	8 ml
2½ fluid drams	—	10 ml
4 fluid drams	—	15 ml
1 fluid ounce	—	30 ml
1¾ fluid ounces	—	50 ml
3½ fluid ounces	—	100 ml
7 fluid ounces	—	200 ml
8 fluid ounces	—	250 ml
1 pint	—	500 ml (approximate)
1 quart	—	1000 ml (approximate)
1 gallon	—	4000 ml (approximate)

CONVERSION TABLE: HOUSEHOLD MEASUREMENTS AND METRIC EQUIVALENTS

1 drop	—	0.06 ml
1 teaspoonful	—	4.0 ml
1 tablespoonful	—	15 ml
1 ounce	—	30 ml
1 cup	—	250 ml
1 pint	—	500 ml (approximate)
1 quart	—	1000 ml (approximate)
1 gallon	—	4000 ml (approximate)

CONVERSION TABLE: POUNDS AND METRIC EQUIVALENTS

1 lb —	.45 kg	45 lbs —	20.5 kg
2 lbs —	.9 kg	50 lbs —	22.7 kg
3 lbs —	1.4 kg	55 lbs —	25.0 kg
4 lbs —	1.8 kg	60 lbs —	27.3 kg
5 lbs —	2.3 kg	65 lbs —	29.6 kg
6 lbs —	2.7 kg	70 lbs —	31.8 kg
7 lbs —	3.2 kg	75 lbs —	34.1 kg
8 lbs —	3.6 kg	80 lbs —	36.4 kg
9 lbs —	4.1 kg	85 lbs —	38.7 kg
10 lbs —	4.5 kg	90 lbs —	40.9 kg
15 lbs —	6.8 kg	95 lbs —	43.2 kg
20 lbs —	9.1 kg	100 lbs —	45.4 kg
25 lbs —	11.4 kg	125 lbs —	56.8 kg
30 lbs —	13.6 kg	150 lbs —	68.1 kg
35 lbs —	15.9 kg	175 lbs —	79.5 kg
40 lbs —	18.2 kg	200 lbs —	90.8 kg

CONVERSION TABLE: FAHRENHEIT THERMOMETER READINGS AND CENTIGRADE EQUIVALENTS

Fahrenheit	Centigrade	Fahrenheit	Centigrade
98.0	36.7	102.4	39.1
98.2	36.8	102.6	39.2
98.4	36.9	102.8	39.3
98.6	37.0	103.0	39.4
98.8	37.1	103.2	39.5
99.0	37.2	103.4	39.6
99.2	37.3	103.6	39.8
99.4	37.4	103.8	39.9
99.6	37.6	104.0	40.0
99.8	37.7	104.2	40.1
100.0	37.8	104.4	40.2
100.2	37.9	104.6	40.3
100.4	38.0	104.8	40.4
100.6	38.1	105.0	40.6
100.8	38.2	105.2	40.7

101.0	38.3	105.4	40.8
101.2	38.4	105.6	40.9
101.4	38.5	105.8	41.0
101.6	38.6	106.0	41.1
101.8	38.7	108.0	42.2
102.0	38.8	110.0	43.3
102.2	39.0		

To convert Fahrenheit thermometer readings into Centigrade:
Subtract 32, multiply by 5, then divide by 9

$$°C = \frac{(°F - 32) \times 5}{9}$$

To convert Centigrade thermometer readings into Fahrenheit:
Multiply by 9, divide by 5, then add 32.

$$°F = \frac{(°C \times 9)}{5} + 32$$

Index

(Names in boldface are major articles. The numerical listing in bold-face indicates the page(s) of each major article.)

345

Ø

More SIGNET Medical Books

☐ **HELP FOR YOUR ARTHRITIS AND RHEUMATISM: All the Facts Your Doctor Doesn't Have Time to Tell You by Dr. Arthur Freese.** Your best home guide to the different kinds, causes and cures—including the very latest medical breakthroughs. (#E8290—$1.75)

☐ **THE SILENT DISEASE: HYPERTENSION by Lawrence Galton, with an Introduction by Frank A. Finnerty Jr., M.D., Chief, Cardiovascular Research, D.C. General Hospital.** Doctors who have researched the #1 cause of heart attack and stroke take you beyond *Type A Behavior and Your Heart* to show you how to save your life! (#J7914—$1.95)

☐ **WHY ME? What Every Woman Should Know About Breast Cancer to Save Her Life by Rose Kushner.** Revised and updated. Here is the book that tells you everything about what nobody likes to talk about—and every woman owes it to herself to know! (#E7692—$2.50)

☐ **OH, MY ACHING BACK: A Doctor's Guide to Your Back Pain and How to Control It by Leon Root, M.D., and Thomas Klernan.** Introduction by James Nicholas, M.D., physician to the N.Y. Jets. Are backaches interfering with everything you do? Here is positive relief for you and tens of millions of Americans with back miseries. This wonderful, long-needed book tells you how you can free yourself of back problems—forever! (#E9396—$2.50)

☐ **THE CHANGING YEARS: The Menopause Without Fear by Madeline Gray.** A book which discusses menopause frankly and sensibly—answers your intimate questions and dismisses your fears with sound arguments and practical suggestions. (#J8429—$1.95)

Buy them at your local

bookstore or use coupon

on next page for ordering.

SIGNET Health Books of Interest

☐ **HOW TO TRIPLE YOUR ENERGY by Leonard Haimes, M.D., and Richard Tyson, M.D.** The doctors' new, easy, and effective program for increasing your vigor and zest. You will be astounded at the amount of energy that can be yours as this easy-to-follow, tested program charts your way to increased vitality and a dynamic, fully productive way of life.
(#E7998—$1.75)

☐ **LIVING SALT FREE AND EASY by Anna Houston Thorburn with Phyllis Turner.** The first specific guide to medically-approved low sodium foods for those who want to live to eat as well as eat to live. Includes a sizable collection of recipes that tastes too good to be diet food!
(#W7120—$1.50)

☐ **THE DIETER'S COMPANION: A Guide to Nutritional Self-Sufficiency by Nikki and David Goldbeck.** Choose the diet that is best suited to you with this essential guide written by two nutrition experts. Included are evaluations of all the well-known diet programs in addition to information on designing your own diet according to your weight, health, and particular food preferences. (#E8783—$2.50)

☐ **THE SUPERMARKET HANDBOOK: Access to Whole Foods by Nikki and David Goldbeck.** This book will prove invaluable to any shopper concerned with the quality and nutritive value of foods available in today's supermarkets. It will help you to understand labels and select foods with a discerning eye, and provides easy, low-cost ways of preparing and using whole foods to replace processed foods. "An enormously useful and heartening work!"*The New York Times*
(#E9635—$2.95)

☐ **YOGA FOR AMERICANS by Indra Devi.** A complete six-week home course in the widely recognized science that offers its practitioners a vital and confident approach to the pressures and tensions of modern living. (#J8530—$1.95)

Buy them at your local

bookstore or use coupon

on next page for ordering.